All Health's Breaking Loose:

The Handbook

by Loa Blasucci

Your personal boot camp guide to becoming your authentic, lean, naturally beautiful self.

Outskirts Press, Inc.
Denver, Colorado

The opinions expressed in this manuscript are solely the opinions of the author and do not represent the opinions or thoughts of the publisher. The author has represented and warranted full ownership and/or legal right to publish all the materials in this book.

All Health's Breaking Loose
A Personal Bootcamp Experience
All Rights Reserved.
Copyright © 2010 Loa Blasucci
V4.0

This book may not be reproduced, transmitted, or stored in whole or in part by any means, including graphic, electronic, or mechanical without the express written consent of the publisher except in the case of brief quotations embodied in critical articles and reviews.

Outskirts Press, Inc.
http://www.outskirtspress.com

ISBN: 978-1-4327-4455-7

Library of Congress Control Number: 2010925302

Outskirts Press and the "OP" logo are trademarks belonging to Outskirts Press, Inc.

PRINTED IN THE UNITED STATES OF AMERICA

Table of Contents

Week 1..13

Week 2..35

Week 3..59

Week 4..89

Week 5..115

Week 6..143

Week 7..159

Appendix
    Let's Begin..189
    Food Journal...193
    Recipes..199
    Acknowledgements...225

Introduction

This program is about you! Your body and your life have brought you to the very place where you are at this moment. Only you know how it has felt to come through the events of your life with the body you have. How do you feel? Are you joyful, lively, strong, and calm? If you carry extra weight, have fatigue or past regrets, if you're just not feeling as good as you used to, or feel like you're getting "old," your body is begging you for help. It's time to feel vital, and glow with inner peace and beauty. In order to move forward from where you're at right now, we need to understand some things about you. Then and only then will your perspective adjust and allow you to move forward with new goals. You don't have to be overweight, out of shape, depressed, or feel older than your age. Whatever your shape and size at this moment, you can feel and look better than you ever have, with renewed energy. You get one body to take you on life's journey and whether that began 20, 30, 40 or 50 plus years ago, your body now tells the story of the emotional and physical trip it has been on. But, you are in charge now. You can be free of the emotional shackles that have bound you to destructive habits such as food addictions, over eating, becoming more and more out of touch with your own body and closing off from the joy and love that is around you. You deserve to be lean, strong, beautiful, and happy. This is your time. Right now.

I live and work in the town of "beautiful people" and was given the opportunity to groom some of the biggest stars and presumably most gorgeous men and women of all time. As a make up artist, working closely with actors, I listened carefully to my clientele. I taught skin care, eating habits, and lifestyle. I disguised flaws and generously highlighted loveliness, which seemed like magic to people. But, observing those sitting in my makeup chair, as I chose from an arsenal of secret weapons neatly packed in my trusted makeup case, I could see the real magic didn't come from me or my tricks. Years of "close-up" examination proved that there was a certain glow that could not be purchased or applied. Rather it was a change that washed over them as they began to look better and feel better about themselves. This "brightness" from the inside seemed to radiate out. No makeup artist or even surgeon can apply it. I became convinced that you don't have to be one of the "beautiful people" to be beautiful.

Authentic beauty has nothing to do with cultural standards for height, weight, or bone structure. Authentic beauty emerges as we learn to embrace and nurture the vitality of a liberated and healthy self. Health, fitness, and emotional wellness are beautiful!

Health and fitness research has been a lifelong passion for me. And as a sports nutritionist and makeup artist, it feels comfortable and natural for me to have a foot planted in both fields. I see them as one industry.

I began putting this program into action with carefully controlled studies in 2002 working one-on-one with clients wanting to change their bodies. With excellent results, I watched clients feel younger and grow leaner. I moved to a group setting with the beginning of my Wellness Boot Camp in 2006, running camps three and four sessions per year. With continued success I have seen this program change more than bodies. It changes lives.

This book is a manual. It is meant to take you on your own personal boot camp journey — to the Authentic You. It is filled with questions that need to be pondered and considered, so keep a pen handy. There is room for journaling and assignments to complete for each week. Rather than chapters, it is broken up into "Weeks" and each section requires about seven days. Stay with each chapter for that amount of time and reread and reconsider your answers before moving on. When we understand you and what you have been through, then we'll know how you got to this place. Then, we can chart a new course. You know your body better than anyone else and the intelligence within you knows how to slow down the aging process, feel content, lose weight, and have a strong and sculpted body protected from disease.

Let's get past all the half-truths of fitness and wellness. The world is a quagmire of health and beauty contradictions. Let's prepare the way so the truth about your body will resonate within you. You will recognize it when your body begins to feel younger. When you feel new energy flowing through you, you'll know you've found your true, authentic path. Your body will surprise you with results you may have never imagined. This program makes this possible. I have seen it happen over and over again.

Steve McQueen's Dog Has a Glass Eye

I love this town! In Los Angeles, name-dropping is normal and commonplace. If you're waiting in line at the market and the guy in front of you wearing a hat looks like Brad Pitt, well, it's probably Brad Pitt, and later you might mention to a

Introduction

friend you saw him. But, in order to keep the focus on you, what follows will be the last of the name-dropping in this book.

When we were kids, my friend was riding her mini bike in the hills of Malibu. She took a fall. As she collected herself, a guy on a motorcycle stopped and called to her to see if she was okay. When she realized it was Steve McQueen — the hottest guy in the universe (it was the sixties) she was thrilled. The next morning at school, she whispered to her friend at the desk next to hers that she "had seen Steve McQueen yesterday in Malibu while riding." Her friend told the student in front of her what had happened, and he told the student across from him, who then told the student next to her and the information made its way across the room. Right before the teacher walked in, the kid farthest away in the corner desk shouted, "What? Steve McQueen's dog has a glass eye?"

And so goes the American fitness industry: a friend tells you that following "this" food plan will help you lose 5 pounds per week. Then your neighbor says, "Yes, but buy these protein drinks." Then one of the trainers at the gym tells you to take kick boxing rather than spinning and a late night infomercial wants you to take supplements and before you know it someone yells, "Steve McQueen's dog has a glass eye!"

Since more than 90 million Americans have a chronic illness — hypertension, arthritis, heart disease, depression, asthma, etc. — and 64 percent of us are

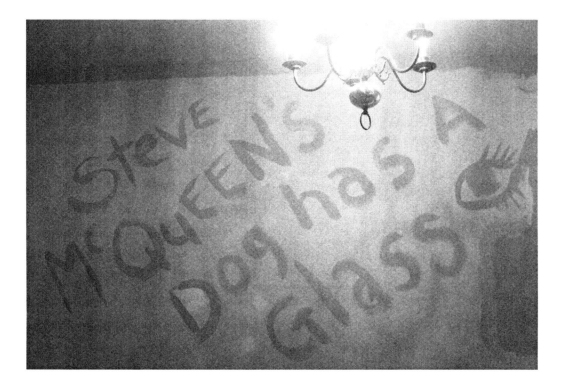

overweight or obese, it begs the question: are we getting the truth? The more toxic we become as a nation, the more obsessed we are with celebrities. The students got Mr. McQueen's name right. Likewise, some of what you've heard about health, fitness, and nutrition has merit. But in this program, your body decides what is true and right for you. There is an efficient way to achieve your goals without wasting time and money. I learned from all those years where real beauty comes from and I want to share that with you now.

You have internal wisdom and instinctively know more about your health and body than you realize. Your health is up to you and your ability to identify truth. This is a plan to help you cut through all the hearsay, folklore, gimmicks and sales pitches to find the real and authentic you. It is a natural, science-based, personalized path to strength, power, health, and beauty. No one has lived your life and had your experiences. It takes time to learn new ways of living. It takes time to unlearn what is no longer useful, or perhaps even in the way. Therefore, this program is presented in a manual format for you to engage week by week. Writing about your feelings will help you to see the path that you have traveled. Let's identify how you became who you are, right at this moment. Your journaling will help your emotions take shape so we know what we're dealing with. Then we can find your own true beautiful self.

I am excited to work with you in this process. Let's get started.

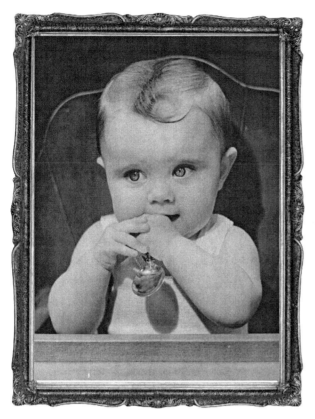

Week 1

This is Where We Begin:
Internal Programming
The "Authentic You"
Storing Emotional Garbage
Hydration

Who Are You — Really?

There you were — a toddler, cruising around the living room in a diaper. I bet you were cute. You listened, you heard, you saw, you took it all in. As a child, you were at your most impressionable. Smaller than your caretakers, you looked up to them, watched how they acted, and listened to their ideas. Your view of the world was taught to you little by little, day by day. For however many years you've been

> This chapter must be confronted and understood before the rest of this program can truly be effective. However, this is not an intellectual exercise. Understanding your emotions is not the same as the willingness to feel them. Take time to acknowledge, ponder and feel. Write to release, then resolve to "let go." This is the first and most important step towards becoming the strong, lean, beautiful person you really are.

alive on this planet, your life training has been unfolding all around you. And here you are now, with the disposition of your body and the feelings of your spirit to show for it.

We are conditioned by events and circumstances that touch our lives. Our observations and experiences — good and bad, happy and sad — shape our attitude and beliefs. Whether or not we're dealing with the truth, our experience creates our awareness. This awareness becomes our reality — our view of the world. It makes us who we are.

The encouragement and the criticism you received from your parents may still run through your mind in the same phrases that were said to you as a child. Some psychologists believe we may receive as many as thirty thousand hours of verbal conditioning from our parents and elders[1]: "Why can't you be like your sister?" "You're so fun to be with." "Hurry up, you're so slow." "He's my shy child." "Why are you so clumsy?"

Think back. What was said to you repeatedly as a child? Record it here.

_____
_____
_____
_____
_____
_____

---

1. Chopra, Deepak. Sacred Verse, Healing Sounds: The Baghavad Gita. New World Library, 2004.

When ideas are drummed into our heads over and over, they become deeply rooted in our psyche. Whether or not they're true, they feel real. These ideas become our perspective and add to our own personal awareness.

We may have as many as 100,000 thoughts in a single day[2]. These thoughts translate into feelings, and those feelings become emotions. Every emotion brings a physical response from the body. Nervousness increases the heart rate and perspiration. Happiness widens the eyes, lifts the delicate face muscles upward, and opens the chest. These reactions happen without conscious effort. Every cell in the body has intelligence and is affected by feelings[3]. Health is directly connected to emotions because the immune system, central nervous system, and endocrine system biologically connect every thought and emotion in your body. For every thought you have, a biological event occurs in your body.

As you journal your answers to these questions, you may have feelings emerge. Recognize these feelings. Be aware of your body's disposition and any changes you may notice as you ponder these memories. Watch for tension or calm that accompanies them. These feelings have created and shaped the physical body that is now "you." Your self-esteem, ambition, disposition, physical capabilities, perseverance, and happiness all stem from learned behaviors, feelings you have been taught. Your life history is stored in your body memory and therefore carried around with you every day, everywhere you go.

How did your mother feel about being a mother?

___

How did your father demonstrate his feelings toward you?

___

Did you feel acceptance as a child?

___

Were you often frightened as a child?

___

Are you content in your current home relationships?

___

___

2. Ishaya, Maharishi Sadashiva. Enlightenment: The Yoga Sutras of Pataniali. Waynesville, North Carolina: SFA Publications, 1996.
3. Chopra, Deepak. Creating Health: How to Wake Up the Body's Intelligence. New York: Vantage Press, 1991.

Stored. Stuck. Shelved. Buried.

All your memories, whether happy or sad, are stored in your body. Getting lost in the grocery store as a child, getting scolded in front of the class by your fourth-grade teacher, scoring the winning touchdown, making the whole class laugh at a funny joke — all are still there. Allowing your body to feel peaceful because of fond memories and keeping your body memory banks free from negative stored emotions are important skills. Trauma from past emotional events may continue to be stressful to the body years after the event has taken place. Your body memory can "re-feel" an event when thoughts return to it or when new circumstances remind you of the old experience. Years after a traumatic event has occurred, your body can experience anxiety, racing heartbeat, sweating, upset stomach, lack of sleep, and many other physical responses from revisiting the event in your thoughts.

> "The sorrow which has no vent in tears may make other organs weep."
> — Henry Maudsley

In time, stored negative emotions can lead to depression, irritable bowel syndrome, chronic anxiety, digestive problems, chronic fatigue, age and frown lines in the face, weight gain from "comfort eating," heart irregularities — the list goes on and on. Stored negative emotions become toxic to all the systems of the body. They do damage on a cellular level and speed up the aging process. They are garbage to your body, and your body is no place to store garbage. Rather, it is the vehicle with which you get to take this journey called life. Your body houses your spirit. It is a gift, and since you are the proprietor of this precious gift, it is your job to keep it clean and pure.

If there are events in your past that elicit physical responses when thinking about them, list them here.

_____
_____
_____
_____
_____
_____

Describe what your emotional status was at the time of those events, and how you feel now as you recall them.

_____
_____
_____
_____
_____
_____
_____

> Alissa was a student of mine. I met with her weekly in her home as she took this program on an individual basis. Her house was huge and immaculate. Maintained sharply in every corner, it looked like a photo in a home design magazine — freshly painted, spotless, every pillow in place. Yet her own personal "house" was full of resentment for an unavailable husband, overflowing with chemicals from the five diet sodas she drank daily, and lacking energy because she ate fast food several times a week. She was overweight, depressed, and guilt-ridden because she had no ambition to exercise. I looked around this incredible house and wondered, *How could the house made of concrete and wood be so much more important than the one that held her spirit, the desires of her heart, her wisdom, her energy — the house that would take her through her entire life?*

We've all been through some things we wish we could have skipped. If you have unresolved pain, fear, resentment, anger, or bitterness stored within you, nothing you read in this book will magically cleanse and heal your body. The process of ridding your body of these toxins begins inside of you. YOU have the power to release this garbage from your body. It may seem like a tall order, but if you want to feel vital, strong, healthy, and beautiful, it has to be done.

The only way to "get it out" is to "go through it." These emotions must be revisited, acknowledged, and understood. No one wants to re-feel trauma, but there is a great purpose in this exercise. It's time to release it and be rid of the suffering forever. Try to find where the distress has been kept inside of you. It may be in soft tissues where you tend to have tension. It may linger as pain and you may notice discomfort in your abdominal area or low back. Maybe it's been held in your upper neck and shoulders, or deep inside in a vital organ.

While you are checking in with your body, analzye the following areas to determine if you have ailments. Really stop and pay attention to what you are feeling.

- ☐ Tightness in the belly
- ☐ Low back pain
- ☐ Neck pain or limited range of motion
- ☐ Shoulder stiffness, pain, or limited range of motion
- ☐ Mid-back pain
- ☐ Aches in the gut and abdominal area
- ☐ All over achiness or lethargy

Feel your way to it — be with the emotion and focus on any lesson you may have learned from this experience. You may have gained compassion, patience, or understanding that otherwise you would not have. You may have gained strength. This is the silver lining.

Please journal all that comes to you surrounding this silver lining.

_____
_____
_____
_____
_____
_____
_____
_____
_____
_____

Because your mind and body are intimately connected, if your heart has been hurt, then so has your body. Psychological and emotional wounding becomes physical. Being beautiful or handsome is not something that just happens to the lucky few — it is determined by a physical, emotional, psychological, and spiritual equation. But your body is an amazing healing machine, and no matter how you feel right now, your body is capable of being more healthy and looking more beautiful than you ever have before. A physical wound — like a cut on your finger — closes itself by forming a scab and a scar, and then, before you know it, the wound is gone. Unlike this physical process, emotional healing begins on the inside by releasing suppressed emotions that have been festering and stagnant. Healing is presumed to happen intellectually. As humans, we know we're smart; we like to collect our personal information and "therapize" ourselves. We like to speculate about why we know what we know. But this life-changing process of healing happens organically in the body as well as in the mind. We can understand the process of healing with our brain, but allowing it to actually happen involves body, mind, heart, and soul.

Tomorrow, read your journaled thoughts, and add any others that have come to you here.

_____
_____
_____
_____
_____
_____

Those "shelved" or "stuffed" emotions are illnesses in the making because they block the flow of your energy. And when those emotions are released, energy is freed and healing powers flow through you. Feelings become genuine because they harbor no bias from your past. Isn't it exciting that we just might learn more about the "Authentic You"? It takes real intention to change your perspective. More than just acknowledging it, you must free yourself from it. Letting go of your early conditioning creates an emotional environment that allows the "Authentic You" to emerge. It allows you to move forward with a more productive and creative lifestyle.

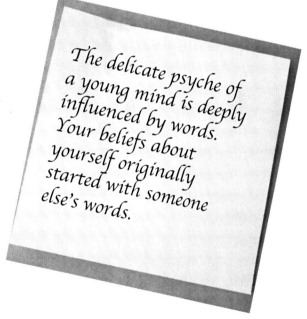

The delicate psyche of a young mind is deeply influenced by words. Your beliefs about yourself originally started with someone else's words.

I wish I knew you and could talk with you about how and why you've held onto these feelings. Maybe it's because the society we live in teaches us to seek control; control is power. We have been taught we must control our emotions, our children and their emotions, and we must not outwardly express those emotions. Or maybe we feel we are not good enough or pretty enough; maybe we have always been the one who takes care of others emotionally, and leaving our own needs last has been a factor. Maybe we feel trapped in a bad situation where we have suffered abuse, either physical or psychological. Whatever the reason for your repressed emotions, now is the time to release these feelings. Let them go, and watch for the wonderful changes in your life — noticeable in your body and face.

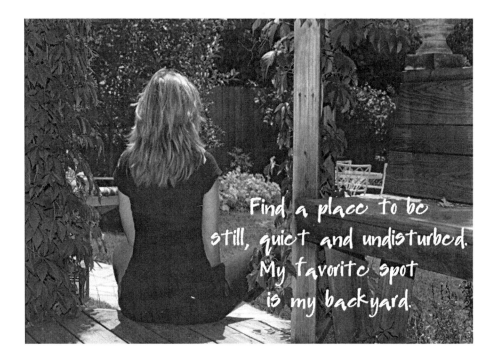

Find a place to be still, quiet and undisturbed. My favorite spot is my backyard.

To truly be rid of stored toxic emotions, you must confront them and sort them out. Think through the events; feel and understand what occurred. This process is not for wimps! It is not easy, but it is imperative and it is truly worth it.

Go to a private place, free of phones and distractions. If you've listed some past events that still create a negative physical response, review them now. Breathe deeply with your eyes closed. If there is sadness, anger, or fear, feel it in your body. If there are tears, let them fall. Listen to your body as you go through this process. Feel where stress is stored and take your awareness to that spot. Listen to your breath. Stay with your feelings. Keep breathing and let go of the pain as you exhale. Visualize this stagnation leaving your body on the breath of each exhale. Stay with this process until you feel clear and released. Know that you will gain health, peace, and beauty from this experience. This is the wisest investment that you can make in your health and longevity.

Journal your experience.

_____
_____
_____
_____

Many will read over this exercise and think, "This is interesting," and brush past it. Others may think, "I am still very vulnerable. Will it be worth it to explore the hurt again?" But it takes wisdom and courage to know there is healing that needs to take place. Dr Deepak Chopra elaborates, "Being hurt isn't pleasant, but it is real. It puts you in the present, whereas conditioned responses of anger, anxiety, guilt, and depression put you out of the present. Once you are in the present you can follow the trail of your emotions back to their source, which is not pain but love, compassion, truth — the real you. There is no purpose in suffering except as a guide to your truth." In this healing process, as you are sorting through the history of events that brought you to where you are at this moment, you will continue to learn about yourself and your body by answering these questions:

1. How did the ideas and attitudes of those around you affect how you dealt with the situation at the time?

_____
_____

2. Can you identify patterns of behavior that stem from the pain?

_____
_____

3. Do you feel your heart is open enough to grow from any life lessons available to you?   Circle YES/NO

Ridding your body of emotions that have been stored for a long time is a process, and it is important to be gentle with yourself as you go through it. Give yourself space; take a break from crowds and busy-ness and avoid contact with difficult or negative people and situations. Rest. Breathe. Drink fresh juices and eat light meals. Take care of yourself. You may experience periods of feeling out of touch, a numbness or fogginess. It is part of your body coming back into balance. Just as your life experiences are uniquely yours, the feelings that emerge for you now may be unique to you as well. The intelligence of your body will eventually get on board and free up blocked energy. You may begin to feel light. Some people experience this light feeling as a "lucky" or "blessed" feeling. Some feel quiet and low-key. Recognize this feeling. Feel it. Listen to your body.

No More Band-Aids

> In 1504, Michelangelo created his masterwork, the Statue of David. He was asked to carve a statue that would stand in the Piazza della Signoria, the town hall of Florence, as a symbol of Florentine freedom. The stone he used was imperfect, but he began the challenge anyway. When asked how he could create such beauty from a piece of stone, he responded, "David was always in there, I just chipped away the excess." We are each in the process of our own "masterwork." It is up to us by way of our choices to chip away the excess around us and let our authentic beauty be revealed. [4]

Regret and anger are toxic to the body. Often these are deeply rooted emotions that stem from a situation, person or idea from which we once had a strong attachment. On a subconscious level, hanging onto the resentment or anger makes us feel that we are still connected to the original situation. Yet we deplete our vitality by storing these emotions.

If regret, fear, bitterness, anger, anxiety, or depression are present in your life, those feelings did not just appear one day out of the blue. Over time, life events — combined with your conditioning — may cause you to look, act, and feel unlike who you really are. Our "microwave society" leads us to believe in the quick and easy fix: "Cover it up. Medicate it. Just fix it fast and make it easy."

Unfortunately, there is no shortcut route that will bypass Week One. And no one else can do it for you — a magical snap of the fingers will not bring you back to square one. This is about finding the "Authentic You." Step by step and thought by thought. You can do this. Let go of any resentment, bitterness, anger, regret, fear, jealousy, anxiety, depression, or other bad feelings, so you can improve your health and feel like your true self.

Mentally picture your body as a white house with white carpet. Angry, resentful, or stressful thoughts are like a muddy rubber kickball ricocheting from wall to wall and floor to ceiling. You can acquire the skills to eliminate these toxic emotions from your mind and, ultimately, from your body. It's time to throw the muddy kickball away.

---

4. University of California Libraries. Michelangelo as a Sculptor. Boston: Bates and Guild, 2007.

As you go through this process, you may catch a glimmer of new blessings. No matter what has happened, those who are wise will learn from their experiences. The greatest learning experience you could have is to find your authentic self. I hope that as some of life's lessons are revealed to you, you can embrace them and keep the wisdom they bring with you always. Good memories aren't always the result of good things. Sometimes we keep good memories because of how we choose to view what happened. You may have more good memories than you think. Be open to finding increased fulfillment in your life and circumstances.

> Everyone's needs are different: listen to your thirst.

H_2O — It's What You're Made Of

This program is about YOU. Right now we're setting up a comprehensive scenario that will bring balance to your body. We can do this through emotional

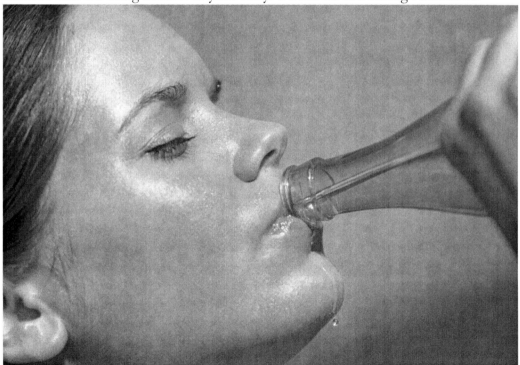

Water — the Fountain of Youth

cleansing, as learned previously, and through physical cleansing. The first step for either one is to keep hydrated.

When the body is in a state of dehydration, it perceives stress. This stress intensifies any imbalance you may already have. We want your body to function with ease so it has surplus energy to heal itself. Staying hydrated is monumentally important, especially right now. If there really were a fountain of youth, water would be the miraculous fluid running through it.

Think about the design of your body. More than 75% of your blood and soft tissue is water, and 85% of your brain tissue is water[5]. Water carries nutrients and oxygen to the cells of your body through the bloodstream. It lubricates the joints, cools the body through perspiration, carries wastes through the body for elimination, and is vital for the chemical reactions of metabolism and digestion. Your small intestine secretes two liters of fluid, which is mostly water, every single day! Without enough water, we would be poisoned to death by our own wastes. You can lose a pint a day just from exhaling, so we even need water to breathe! If all the water were taken out of your body, you could hold the dry remains in your hands.

Dehydration causes poor muscle tone, excess body fat, lethargy, depression, anxiety, and a myriad of other problems. Chapped lips, constipation, dark urine,

> ## Drink it Up
>
> 1. Drink good quality bottled, filtered, 7.0 pH balanced water.
> 2. Drink from glass containers rather than plastic whenever possible.
> 3. Add a slice of lemon and a sprig of fresh mint.
> 4. Drop a mint tea bag in your glass, stir lightly and remove it.
> 5. Freeze lemon juice with a shake of Stevia or agave nectar (these natural sweeteners will not affect your glycemic index) in ice cube trays. Drop one into a tall glass of water.
> 6. Add a splash of chilled herb tea to your water.

---

5. Dr. Allen, Corrine, Ph.D. "Water and the Brain." www.BrainAdvance.org. http: globalkangen.info/Documents/1brainwater.pdf.

and thirst are outward signs of dehydration. When you are dehydrated, your body must "rob Peter to pay Paul," redistributing fluids to take care of the most vital processes, which throws off the balance of your system. Balance and proper hydration are crucial to your health.

One set amount of water will not suit everyone's individual needs. An NBA player requires a different amount than a 5-foot-tall grandmother. The processes of your body are very personally yours, driven by your DNA and the foods you eat. Simply put, some people sweat more than others. Factor in the climate in which you live and how active you are, and you will begin to see that the amount of water you need to drink is continually changing and unique to you. The best guide is to listen to your body, recognize thirst, and be mindful of your needs. Before noon, your body gears up for the day and needs water available, so plan to consume approximately half of your daily water intake before twelve.

If you sweat heavily (with a noticeable perspiration on face, and wet hair during medium exercise), you may use this simple rule to calculate your individual need[6]: Half your body weight in ounces daily. For example, if your body weight is 160 pounds, half of that is 80. Divide 80 ounces by 8 oz. (which is in one cup) = 10 cups. Therefore, 10 cups per day would be required for a person who weighs 160 pounds. This is an approximation — hot, dry weather and exercise raise your daily requirement and each of us have different demands within our own body. It's best to let your body guide you. Be mindful of dryness in the mouth, face, and hands, and keep a running tab — on paper — of the number of 8 oz. glasses you have each day. When you get the hang of how it feels to be hydrated, keep the tab in your head.

> *The illiterate of the 21st century will not be those who cannot read and write, but those who cannot learn, unlearn, and relearn.*
> *— Alvin Toffler*

As a warning for the over-zealous, this is not a situation of "the more the merrier." Drinking too much water taxes the kidneys and gives the body excess work to do, so don't overdo a good thing.

Stay away from "sports drinks" or colored designer waters. Athletic performance is not enhanced by adding sugars or artificial colors to the body. It's the American way, isn't it? Make it sweeter and prettier, and you'll buy a whole lot more of it! But all you purchase is hype and advertising.

6. Covey, Stephen R. "Health & Your Parents." www.usaweekend.com/08_issues/080203/080203health-aging-parents.html. 15 July 2009.

Eliminate carbonated waters and soft drinks, which contain carbon dioxide. To your body, carbon dioxide is garbage — a waste product. By consuming "bubbly" water and soft drinks, you feed your body a waste product — just one more toxin to process. Pure, clean, room temperature water with a pH no lower than 7.0 is the best beverage for the body. A good quality bottled water will list the pH on the label. If it's not listed, chances are it was processed inexpensively and is too acidic for your body. Good water is your fountain of youth.

Monitor your water intake daily. Record it in the chart in Appendix A in the back of the book.

Moving Ahead

If you are confused, feel an internal heaviness, or are still unsure about the work you have done this week, do not move ahead to Week 2. Go back and read from the beginning. Review your journal, adding thoughts where you feel the need. Stay with this week's exercises until you have released the negative emotional energy and feel it is no longer with you. This is your chance to discover what it is like to feel free and strong with brightness in your eyes and enthusiasm for what lies ahead of you. You deserve to be calm and happy with a lean body, glowing skin, and the energy to accomplish whatever you want. This week is where it begins and it can't be rushed. Watch for a feeling of lightness deep from within. Listen to your body, and you will know when it is time to move ahead.

A "Weighty" Issue

Do you remember that old riddle we heard back in the fifth grade, "What weighs more, a pound of feathers or a pound of rocks?" Your first inclination may have been that of course, rocks are heavier than feathers. But the real answer is hidden in the question. This riddle came rushing back to memory one morning as I heard some of my students commiserating after a fitness workshop. They were stressed about their weight and how it continually creeps up. One of them blurted out, "But doesn't muscle weigh more than fat?" I could see in their faces the genuine anxiety many of us have about our weight. Far too many misconceptions exist about the relationship between health and weight. These myths bring fear that causes self-esteem to nose dive.

A cup of fat weighs less than a cup of muscle. To say muscle weighs more than fat is a conundrum: a pound of each weighs, well … a pound. But, muscle is more compact and smooth. It's denser, unlike adipose tissue (fat), which is lumpier and takes up 20% more space than muscle[7]. Muscle and fat look very different on our bodies because of their composition and where we tend to carry them. Fat collects in areas of our bodies that take away definition and shape. You notice it especially in the face and around the midsection. Our number one concern about fat should not be how it looks on our body but rather how it affects its function, vitality, and longevity.

> *A solid body has more muscle mass and more potential for strength.*

One of my first jobs as a young adult was working at the New Life Health Spa. My job was to weigh and measure all new clients and show them how to use the fitness equipment in the gym. I was taking a new client through the routine — I took all her measurements — waist, hips, bust, rib cage, arms, legs, and height. I then realized she was exactly my height and size. We were chatting about our exactness of size as we walked over to the scale. She stepped on and to my surprise, she weighed nine pounds less than I did! This really bothered me. It seemed so unfair — if according to height and size we were identical, why did I have to weigh so much more? I felt cheated. For many years of my life I was embarrassed about how much I weighed. More so than how I looked, it was the number on the scale that bothered me. It always seemed higher than that of my peers and I was ashamed to actually say the number. I have since learned that even though it was a sore spot for years, there was a silver lining.

A solid body has more muscle mass and more potential for strength. Carrying more muscle means you burn more calories throughout the day — as muscle burns 19 times more calories than fat does[8]. Over the years, this translates into many pounds that will not accumulate on your body.

Why is the number on the scale important to you? Maybe having our weight quantified is confirmation that we exist; we take up space and weigh "this much." Maybe the number on the scale makes fitness seem like an exact science. If the

---

7. Novick, Jeff. "Does Muscle Weigh More Than Fat?" National Health Association. 27 April 2009. www.healthscience.org/index.php?option=com_content&view=article&catid=102%3Ajeff-novicks-blog&id=549%3Adoes-muscle-weight-more-than-fat&Itemid=267.
8. "How to Make Your Body Burn More Calories." Weight Loss Resources. 5 July 2009. www.weightlossresources.co.uk/calories/burning_calories/burn_more_calories.htm.

number is low; you are sexy with a good life. The number creeps up and you're hit with a tidal wave of insecurity and self-doubt. Your very character is called into questions. Remember, weight does not determine your size, shape, or health. Though it may be a contributing factor, a more accurate gauge of health and wellness is how you feel.

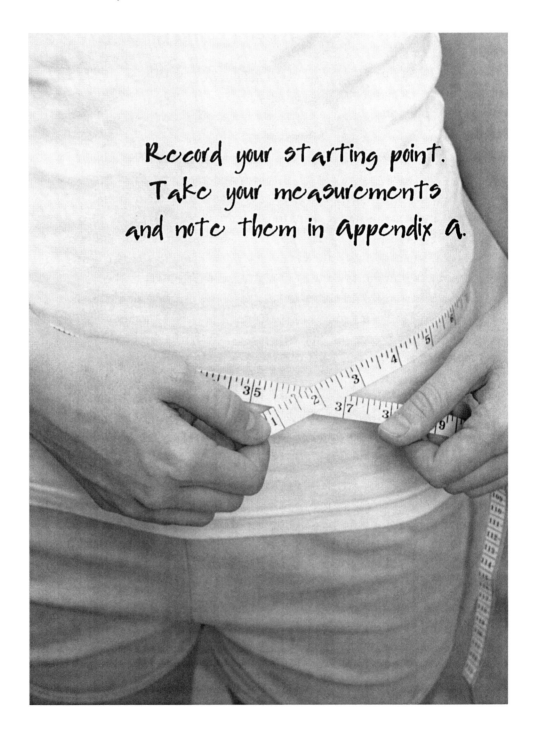

Sometimes, heavier is better. Here are a few things that can add pounds and may enhance your health at the same time.

- Dense bones weigh more and are more resistant to injury and osteoporosis[9].
- Hydration keeps your many systems running, as body fluids circulate throughout your body — in the colon, intestines, joints, and stomach. Your entire body uses fluid for its function. A properly hydrated body may weigh more but handles its functions more efficiently. The skin will have less wrinkles and crepiness, especially in your face.
- Proper long-term exercise distributes muscle mass evenly to the front as well as to the backside of your body. You may not see your backside often but if your exercise routine is balanced, you may have exchanged muscle for fat in places you haven't noticed. This also improves definition and posture.
- The more muscle you carry, the more calories you burn, not just during exercise but 24/7. The more calories you burn, the leaner you stay over time[10].

One of our goals in this program is to release anxiety about issues that don't matter. So let me remove your weight from your list of things to worry about. There's no need to be uneasy about the number of pounds you weigh. What's important is feeling healthy and strong with clothes that hang on your body in a way that makes you feel lean and confident.

Your measurements are a much more accurate gauge of what is happening in your body. I will not ask you to record your weight but we need to document accurate body measurements as you begin this program. Turn to Appendix A and carefully record all the measurements called for. You should wear the same clothing and use the same tape measure each time you take your measurements. If the tape measure is indenting the clothing or skin line, you are pulling too tightly. Allow the tape to lay flat against the skin. Worry more about whether you are smarter than a fifth grader at solving riddles like "what weighs more …" than about the number on the scale.

Getting Started.
You Will Need:

- Probiotics — for internal health and strong intestinal flora. Choose a brand that must be refrigerated. Take one tablet daily starting now.
- Grapefruit seed extract drops — take 10-15 drops stirred into ¼ cup of mangosteen or pomegranate juice daily. Not to be taken at the same time as your probiotic.

---

9. "Bone Mineral Density." Web MD. 5 July 2009. www.webmd.com/_osteoporosis/bone-mineral-density.
10. "How to Make Your Body Burn More Calories." Weight Loss Resources. 5 July 2009. www.weightlossresources.co.uk/calories/burning_calories/burn_more_calories.htm.

- Mini Cleanse — for next week. Find an herbal tablet preparation to assist in cleansing all body systems. Taken with regular meals, it should include blood detoxification, fat metabolizer, hepatic and intestinal factors, and should be prepared to support all organ functions. Shop for a quality cleanse now so you are prepared for next week.
- Good cross training or running shoes and cushioned socks
- Loofah sponge
- Exercise mat
- An organized kitchen with a cutting board and sharp knives for meal preparation.
- "A" list items that we will discuss in a later chapter and lots of amazing, organic fresh foods
- Grapefruit and lavender essential oils (optional)

Note: Grapefruit seed extract and cleansing herbs are not meant for continual use and should be used with caution.

This Week's Assignments:

- Take your probiotic each day.
- Read and sign your personal contract (found on the next page).
- Begin taking your herbal cleanse tablets as recommended.
- Spend a minimum of 20 minutes daily pondering and journaling in this manual.
- Take 10–15 drops of grapefruit seed extract.
- Let go of negative emotions you have been carrying around inside.
- Begin light exercise such as walking, stretching, or gentle yoga — 30 minutes or more daily.
- Avoid any added sugar. More on this to come.
- Calculate your daily requirement for water. Record your water intake each day of the week in the recording log found in Appendix A in the back of the book.
- Record measurements in the recording log found in Appendix A. We will retake your measurements later in the program. Every time you take measurements, make sure to wear the same clothes and use the same tape measure for accuracy.
- Familiarize yourself with the recording log in Appendix A in the back of the book. Not only will you record water intake and measurements every week, but you will also record food intake, meditation, and exercise time.

Camper's Contract

IF you had to put one person in charge of your most treasured possession, what type of person would you choose? Would you want them to be all talk but not motivated? Or, would you trust a person who willingly takes action and does whatever is needed to get the job done? We recognize how important strong leaders are.

TO reach your goals, you need to be a strong leader of yourself. Right now, YOU are the captain of the ship. You are in charge.

THIS program is divided into weeks to allow a smooth transition to an athletic body and a polished fresh face. A quick read-through of this manual will not bring about results. As we go step by step, the transformation begins on the inside, and this takes time. Designate the next 40 days as a time frame to improve your health. Great things can be accomplished in this amount of time. It is important that you

> *When I walk into my kitchen today, I am not alone. Whether we know it or not, none of us is. We bring fathers and mothers and kitchen tables, and every meal we have ever eaten. Food is never just food. It's also a way of getting at something else: who we are, who we have been, and who we want to be.*
> *— Molly Wizenberg*

set aside 90 minutes each day for this essential process. Your health, happiness, and the ability to remain disease-free are important. This is your time to step aside from chronic meaningless events such as ringing phones, TV shows, celebrities' personal problems, noise, and other time wasters and to engage in something truly important: your long-term health.

FOR THE NEXT 40 DAYS YOU ARE IN TRAINING

**If you have a reliable counselor or therapist productively assisting you in pursuit of your wellness, consult with your professional regarding the exercises in this manual. They are designed to work in conjunction with that treatment.

Now is the time to be the leader that can take charge and protect this precious treasure — your health. To ensure you will be true to yourself and your goals, you'll need to be in attendance daily (a quiet place without distractions, with this book in hand). Just showing up is 95% of the challenge. You improve your chances of success greatly by committing to do one thing — show up.

TERMS

1. In order to accomplish my goals I will prioritize my time each day. I will arrange my schedule to have at least 90 minutes each day to dedicate to the challenges in this program. The time that works best for me is the morning/evening from ____am/pm to _____am/pm.
2. I will not calendar an event in place of this time that has been set aside for my personal progress.
3. I realize there is nothing more important for me to be doing at this point in my life — even if it seems more pressing.
4. I will consider this MY time. I feel lucky to have the opportunity to engage in a dynamic personal experience.

I HAVE READ AND UNDERSTAND THESE TERMS.
INITIALS: _____

I, _____ , COMMIT TO PRIORITIZE MY TIME BEGINNING TODAY UNTIL _____ (40 DAYS FROM NOW). I WILL BE ON TIME AT _____ AM/PM AND READY FOR TRAINING. I WILL SMILE AND BE POSITIVE TOWARDS MYSELF AND THOSE AROUND ME. I UNDERSTAND THE IMPORTANCE OF SHOWING UP.

SIGNED_____

DATE_____

When you find yourself stepping out of your comfort zone and trying even though you are afraid, that is when you gain confidence and personal power.

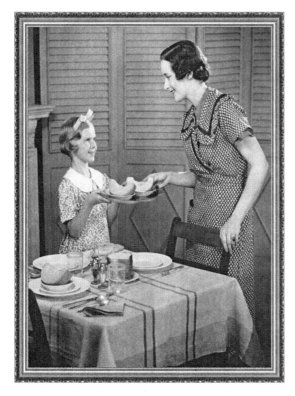

Week 2

This Week's Focus:

Eliminate Toxins
Eat for Vitality
Meditation
Personal Awareness

Starting From the Inside Out

    Energy is not only in every cell of our body, but in everything on this planet — both around us and through us. How we use our own energy, and how we respond to the energy around us, determines our personal rate and process of aging. Whether you are a working individual in a high-stress job, a stay-at-home parent in charge of a household, or you are coming in to a new phase of your life, you are constantly in exchange with the busy world around you. There will be conflicts and exchanges that aren't always uplifting, and as you feel internally — you react outwardly.

In any situation, you can consider the impact of your body's reactions by asking: *Has this experience left me with "less" or "more"?* A "more" experience leaves you with more confidence, more happiness, more growth and more health, even if on a subconscious level. A "more" experience allows the body and mind to stay at peace. A "less" experience is toxic to the body and mind. It leaves you feeling "less" than you are — less healthy, less fulfilled, less loving, and less capable. A "less" experience could be a resentment that is stored inside, or an emotion — once felt deeply — that was buried or hidden away. Still a part of your psyche and lingering in the soft tissues of the body, these old, stagnant emotions deplete your energy, "brightness," and enthusiasm. Conversely, finding the life lesson in an experience proves it to be a "more" experience, even if at first it felt like "less." If you continue to learn from these experiences you will have the ability to feel "more" in your life no matter what the circumstances.

Since emotions dictate much of your health and aging process, it's easy to understand that your face reacts to what you feel. The emotional events happening on the inside of your body become visible in your face.

Anger brings a stiffness or hardness to the face: furrowing the brow (when angry or focusing the eyes) causes wrinkling in the forehead and lowering in the brow. This makes the face appear heavier and the eyes less expressive. Anger may also create tiny broken capillaries around the nose and cheeks. People — particularly women — who store resentment, bitterness, or sadness are more prone to jowling, sagging around the jawline, undereye puffiness, and heavy nasolabial folds (the line that runs from the corner of the nose to the side of the mouth).

Sadness and hopelessness often lead to low energy and low motivation — seen on our faces as a lack of muscle tone. A person with depression may have an oxygen-starved body. As time passes, this lack of cell-rejuvenating oxygen will bring crepiness, or fine crackling lines, to the skin. Over time, "less" emotions leave the face dull and without its glow because emotional energy is tied up storing negative emotions and eliminating a healthy flow.

> Maren was a dear friend and classmate of mine in high school. She was tall, beautiful, and fun-loving. After we graduated, I moved to another state and we lost touch for several years. Then I ran into a friend who had Maren's phone number, so I called her. We had a long visit on the phone and she opened up about her home life during our teenage years, a subject that she had always

kept a secret. Her father had been physically abusive to her. He had been angry because of her sister's unwanted pregnancy, and he took it out on Maren in the form of serious beatings. She left home and married a man who also was abusive to her. He wouldn't allow her privacy and sexually assaulted her. She was still with him, living in a constant state of fear. We made a point to get together in a couple of weeks when I would be in town. When I saw her I couldn't believe my eyes. A woman in her 30s, she looked old enough to be my mother. Her face was weathered and lined, the light in her eyes gone. She was unrecognizable as the Maren I once knew. The toxic effect of living in fear and sadness for so many years was evident in her chalky, weathered face.

We all change in appearance as we progress in life, but the change in Maren was not natural. Where had my friend gone?

We create our own beauty through the choices we make. If there are lines in your face that bother you, describe them here and the emotion you feel that causes them. What event in your life brings this emotion with it?

_____
_____
_____
_____
_____
_____
_____
_____
_____
_____

Toxins come in all shapes and sizes. Some have been packaged, dressed up, hyped up, and marketed to appear beneficial to us. Some continue to pop into our lives through relationships we create or are born with — yes, this could mean family members or friends. We need to honestly consider the effect that each toxin has on us, whether they are in the form of foods, substances, relationships, or feelings.

Have the intention to stay free. There is no greater beauty treatment than cleansing the body. Make a decision to eliminate all toxins from your life. It is up to your good judgment to realize who and what to eliminate.

- On a scale of 1-10, rate how you feel about your weight — 10 means you are confident about the way you look, and are the size and weight you'd like to be, and 1 means your physical appearance brings you sadness and lowers your own self image.

    1   2   3   4   5   6   7   8   9   10

- Circle the foods you crave or have compulsion to eat, drink or "use":

    coffee   breads   diet soda
    soda   salty foods   sweets
    alcohol   chocolate   fast food
    fried foods   cigarettes   other: _____

- Collectively rate the relationships in your life — 10 means they are fullfilling and peaceful, and 1 means they are difficult, strained, or bothersome.

    1   2   3   4   5   6   7   8   9   10

- Rate how much you worry — 10 means you worry to the point of nervousness and anxiety, and 1 means you have a nearly constant state of calm, peacefulness, and happiness.

    1   2   3   4   5   6   7   8   9   10

My worries or negative repeating thoughts are usually about

_____

_____

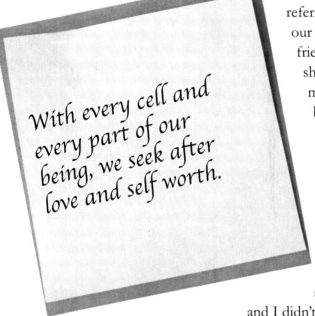

With every cell and every part of our being, we seek after love and self worth.

Barbara was referred to me through our mutual hairdresser friend. He recommended she see me for a make-up consultation because of her recent cosmetic surgery. She was friendly and anxious to learn how to enhance her new, very different face. Barbara was 55 years old with a manicured exterior and I didn't want our time together to be only about the appearance of her face. Her consultation lasted about three hours and during this time she decided she would like to explore more about how her body and face got to the place they were at. She began this program and I knew our first order of business would be her caffeine addiction. She was hyper-attentive and jittery, with her thoughts all over the place. She was "lit" — doing the Starbucks dance as so many Americans do. Barbara was in the clutches of a 10-cups-of-coffee-per-day habit. I made some recommendations and she tried them, but I could see the addiction still had her.

During our fourth meeting, Barbara could barely speak as she expressed feelings about her father. As a child, her father basically ignored her. Absent frequently, he was a man of few words — except during their morning coffee. He loved to make coffee in the kitchen, and she would sit at the table and try to visit with him while they had coffee together. This was the only time he ever spoke to her. I could feel the tenderness of the memory as her tears fell and dampened her blouse.

Barbara was not only dealing with a physical addiction to caffeine, but she also had a very strong emotional attachment to coffee. Her life had trained her to believe that having coffee was a nurturing and rewarding experience for her. However, caffeine was breaking down her body, and emotionally it masked her longing for an attentive father's love. The two toxins were intertwined or "piggybacking."

As she carefully embraced this program, Barbara came to terms with her feelings about her dad. She now has a cup or two of decaffeinated coffee daily and enjoys lots of herb teas as well. The ritual is still very important to her. She has outfitted herself with distinctive tea pots, beautiful mugs, and nurturing aromas to help her feel the ceremony she loved as a child. She constantly searches for a wonderful new tea and has a newfound sense of authentic enjoyment for this ritual in her life.

Since our motives (supporting the family, feeding the kids) don't feel "bad" to us, they create a place for an addiction to settle in or even hide. Because of what we "believe" (we should be a good provider or good nurturer) we set out to fulfill these desires. The overworking, overeating, sugar addiction, alcoholism, or gambling just happens to find its "purposeful" existence in our lives.

- Feeding small children three square meals a day means lots of cooking and eating with the kids — when in fact you may not have been hungry. Caring for and eating with the kids is "good," yet somehow you find yourself eating more than you need.

- Being the breadwinner means hard work is "good," so how can "overworking" be bad?

One of our first instincts at birth is to eat, and that impulse continues many times a day for the rest of our lives. And most likely, many of the emotional events in our lives include food. We attach importance to the food rather than the events — "after-dinner drink," "birthday cake," "afternoon snack," "comfort food," "Sunday dinner." Food attachments weigh us down physically and mentally. They not only alter our physical bodies but our perspectives as well. Remember, we have two things to work with throughout the course of our lives — one is our DNA and the other is our perspective. We must never underestimate the power of perspective. Addiction to a toxic food or substance is not something we "have." If you are addicted, then this toxin "has" you. It has you because you perceive it (physically or emotionally) to be more important than it is critical.

Is there a food or beverage that you bring into your body habitually? Do you feel it is an addiction? Journal about when it began, how it makes you feel and how it affects your life.

_____
_____
_____
_____
_____
_____

Food addictions affect every aspect of our well-being. They are common and often go unattended because we mask or ignore the effects they have on us. We may not even realize we have them because they can "piggyback" or be hidden behind other behaviors.

It was my good fortune to have as a student the most ornery and cantankerous woman I have ever met, simply because I learned so much in dealing with her. Pam was in her late 30s. She wasn't speaking to her father or her siblings. Most of her co-workers avoided her, but she said she didn't care because she didn't need them anyway. She spoke with a bossy, snappy tone in her voice. Once, in a strangely fond way, she referred to her son as a "complete moron."

As I listened to her views on life and the world around her, her health problems didn't surprise me. Her "prickly" disposition had set the tone in her body. She had limited flexibility in her body, redness from burst capillaries in her face, painful bone spurs (calcium deposits in her foot), and a recently abnormal pap smear. Emotionally she was toxic.

There was no available energy to heal these problems as they manifested themselves. Her body was breaking down. Pam was willing to make a few dietary adjustments, which improved her health moderately, but she has continued to struggle with letting go of some past resentments that keep her anger burning. Sometimes we hang on tightly to anger because it is familiar, and not knowing what we would have left in its place is frightening.

Our bodies speak to us in many ways. They give us direction. It is our job to learn to listen to the wisdom of our bodies.

Is your body telling you something about the relationships in your life? Do you carry anger towards someone? Journal who and why and how long you have held on to this anger or resentment.

_____
_____
_____
_____
_____
_____

Does this anger or resentment bring physical symptoms?

_____
_____

Listen for the Ticking

It was harvest time, and the farmer was busily working in the barn. He reached into his pocket for his watch and realized it was gone. His grandfather had given him the watch, and it was his treasure. He quickly called out for his field hands to come into the barn and help him look for it. They frantically combed the barn over, bumping into one another, restacking the hay and searching every square inch of the barn. Exhausted, they found nothing. Finally, the dejected farmer gave

> Many thoughts and feelings have made you who you are. Chronic over-thinking ages the body and face by increasing perceived stress and reducing healing energy.

up and went into the house where he sat with his face in his hands. A few minutes later, his young son came in with an outstretched arm and he slowly opened his fingers. There in the palm of his chubby hand was the watch. The farmer was so excited he hugged the boy and said, "Oh, thank you, son. How on earth did you find it?" The young boy responded, "When the barn was quiet, I could hear the watch ticking."

Creating Internal Peace

We have fast food, internet shopping, cell phones, and laptops. People speed down the road to be on time to yoga class so they can calm down. This "microwave" world is full of words, numbers, and noise. The noise and technological advancements, supposed to make things easier, have actually created a faster paced environment that keeps the mind in a constant state of hyperactivity, or "monkey mind." Thoughts racing, layering on top of each other, bouncing around so fast it becomes hard to focus — it's as if there were a nervous monkey in there jumping around. What a blessing it is to have the skills to release this burden from the mind. Meditation will soothe this nervous monkey.

Time spent meditating is an investment in your health. Meditation has been proven scientifically to improve healing in stress-related conditions. Since 85 percent of visits to a general practitioner's office in the United States are due to stress-related illness, there is much to be gained by practicing meditation[1]. Meditation has been effective in treating high blood pressure, insomnia, PMS, depression, anxiety, and even injuries. It keeps the mind sharp and wards off dementia and memory loss.

The mind replenishes itself through meditation. All things in nature operate in cycles and rhythms of activity and rest. If the mind stays in a state of activity all the time, there is too much energy being spent and not enough being gained. Personal rewards, such as creativity, love, intuition, and stability, can be found in silence through our awareness.

---

1. Randolphi, Ernesto A. Ph. D. Outcomes of Preventive Health Programs Conference December 12–13, 1996. Atlanta, Georgia. Research on Clinical Effectiveness of Stress Management.

Learning to become mindful will replace toxic emotions with peace, intuition, and awareness. This helps to release the desire for a toxic habit, food, or emotion. The practice of meditation brings the ability to live in the present moment. When you are in the present moment, your body energy is not tied up in past hurts and regrets, nor is it tied up in worries and anxieties about the future. Instead, this vital energy becomes available to heal and rebuild the body. Therefore, in the present moment you have no problems. You notice a sense of real joy that comes from deep within you. Contemplation puts you in touch with your true feelings, bringing you insights to where harmony and fulfillment are lacking in your life — it is a beauty treatment for the body and soul.

My profession for 30 years was to search for the finest, most cutting-edge facials and beauty treatments in the world. Many actresses I worked with wanted the best; cost was no factor. But even with the best products available, there is no facial on the market that can bring the relaxed glow to the face as meditation practice does.

Meditation involves going inward to be with and understand the "Authentic You." It requires spending 25–30 minutes a day being still, introspective, and open. This is where many people decide, "Well that's just not for me." "It's too hard," "too time consuming," or "I have too much to do." You may have had thoughts like these, but I will tell you this: when you allow your body and mind to work in synergy, it is more than worth it. Take the opportunity to improve your health and life.

I had some spider veins in my upper thigh that had bothered me for a few years. In the spring, I decided it was finally time to find out about having have them removed. They were painful as well as unsightly. I took a good look at them and called a highly recommended dermatologist to make an appointment. She was booked for about six months. I was a little disappointed but figured it had to be done, so I scheduled the appointment and waited.

> *Just as concentration improves brain power and cognitive function, the practice of releasing racing thoughts fortifies and exercises the brain.*

It was during this time that I learned to meditate, and I began the fitness program that I now teach. The following autumn, six months later, as I looked through my day planner, I noticed that my appointment to see this doctor was the following week. At that moment I looked down at my leg and the red veins were gone. I twisted around to see the backs of my legs, checked my ankles, calves, everywhere, and they were simply gone. No sign of them. I knew exactly where they had been and what they looked like so I was perplexed.

Listen and feel

A few weeks later, I was scheduled to have my annual eye exam. I have my eyes checked every year in the same optometrist's office, by the same doctor. They have a photo on file of the back of my eyes to monitor the macula over time. This exam showed my vision had improved by 10 points! The doctor was surprised — I was at the age where he expected to see a decline in my vision, rather than an improvement.

There are a myriad of other things in my body that have markedly improved since I began to meditate. I was just amazed when I noticed these things, and finally it occurred to me that my body was healing itself. I hadn't consciously tried to correct these things, but the intelligence of my body knew they needed attention. Meditation had brought my awareness to a new level, and without even thinking about this process, healing had taken place. The intelligence of my body was at work — without my being conscious of it. Meditation had brought me such a bonus.

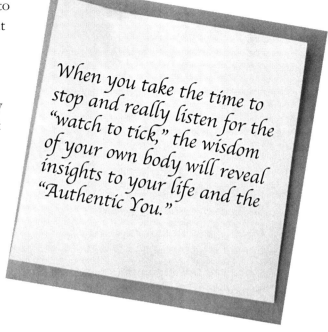

When you take the time to stop and really listen for the "watch to tick," the wisdom of your own body will reveal insights to your life and the "Authentic You."

I wish I could be there with you to discuss your feelings about meditation. What experiences have you had with meditation? Are you eager and willing, or anxious and apprehensive? You will have to be your own guide to understanding this process because there are many ways to approach meditation. It is your most effective tool in mind/body integration. When the mind and body are working together in synergy, the body heals itself more efficiently, and you become in tune with the functions and processes of your body. Stress and aging processes are halted. Your creative process awakens and brings you happiness in ways that will surprise you. Meditation teaches you the language of your body, and when you are in tune with your body, health and beauty are yours. It begins by being conscious of your breath. You breathe approximately 25,000 times a day, 17 times per minute — but how many of those breaths are you aware of? Just being still and noticing your breath will begin the meditation process.

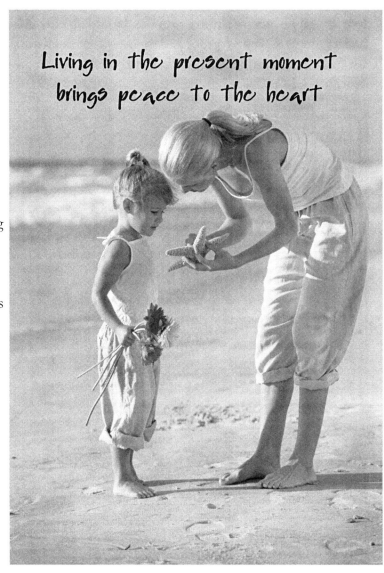

Living in the present moment brings peace to the heart

Remember, this is personal. You can choose the place, the time of day that's most convenient, and whether you sit or lie down — it's all up to you. Try an approach that appeals to you. There are many methods and styles, and I will offer some guidelines:

---

2. Respiratory Health, March 19, 2007. Department of Health and Human Services. 25 July 2009. www.womenshealth.gov/pub/the-healthy-woman/respiratory_health.pdf.

Meditation and your Diet

Meditation enhances the desire to eat a wholesome diet. I have seen clients lose several pounds, often five or more, by adding only meditation to their life. Maintaining a feeling of peace and wellness creates less desire to eat and a craving for foods that bring health and vitality. You will begin to WANT what it is that you actually NEED. This is balance.

> ### Meditation Guidelines:
> 1. Set aside a time daily, preferably 20 to 30 minutes.
>
> 2. Find a quiet, undisturbed place of your choice — a comfortable chair, a spot in your garden, your patio, the beach or wherever you will be able to find quiet.
>
> 3. Unplug. Make sure cell phone, TV and radios are turned off. Put a "do not disturb" sign on the door if necessary.
>
> 4. You may want to tip your head forward slightly, and close your eyes to "shut out" any outside distractions.
>
> 5. Do not meditate when your stomach is full, or if you are hungry.
>
> 6. Use the upcoming meditation as often as you need until you have it in your memory.

Try This

Begin abdominal breathing. Think of a little baby lying on his side in his crib, and notice how his belly rises and falls as he breathes in and out. Focus on your belly. Let it rise as you breathe in and fall as you exhale. Listen to the sound of your breath.

Starting with the feet, point both toes as far as you can, holding it until have you drawn in a long full breath. As you exhale, release the feet. Rest a moment. Flex the feet, drawing the toes up towards your knees as you draw in another long full breath. Release them as you exhale. Rest a moment.

Take your awareness to your glutes; squeeze them as you breathe in. This may elevate you a little. Tighten your rear end and draw in a slow, full breath. Then, as you exhale, release the tightness. Rest a moment.

Extend the fingers on both hands as far apart as possible, as if you were trying to reach one more key on the piano. Press them out, extending your thumb and little finger as far apart as you can get them. Take a deep breath, and as you exhale, release the hands. Rest a moment.

Next, lift both shoulders. Squeeze them up, hold it for a second or two as you are breathing in, and set them down as you let the breath go.

Lastly, tighten the muscles in your face without scrunching or wrinkling the skin. Purse your lips as the skin over the cheek bones tightens smoothly. Raise your brows and lift your ears, holding them taut as you breathe in. Release them gently as you exhale. Return to your breath.

Focus now on the inside of your body. Visualize all the organs of your body, being aware of all they do every minute of the day to keep your body functioning. Stop at each one to thankfully acknowledge it and its capability. Feel appreciation for your body. Keep the breath coming in and out of your belly. Feel the air on your skin.

Be mindful of the energy that is all around you, running through you, and in every single thing on this planet. Feel it holding you together, lifting you upward.

With this next breath, take your awareness to something you have inside that you do not need in your life: resentment, anger, bitterness, or fear. Focus on what it is. Then, as you draw in a slow, full breath, send that stored emotion out of the body with the breath. Feel your body, see if you can feel where it releases from.

For the next few breaths, try to extend the amount of time it takes you to exhale so that it is longer than the time it takes you to inhale. If you can, count slowly in your mind to 3 as you inhale, then count slowly to 4 as you exhale. On the next breath, count to 3 again on the inhale and then to 5 on the exhale. Next, breathe in, count to 3, and then count to 6 as you exhale, if you can.

Take your awareness to what it is that you need in your life. Is it love, peace, joy, fun, beauty? Whatever it is, focus on that concept. As you draw in the next full breath, bring it in to every corner, every place in your body, down to your toes and out to your hands, up to the inside of your head. Draw that emotion into your body, and rather than think about it, bring that positive emotion in to the body with the breath. Stay with your breath; listen to it. Feel the weightlessness of your body. Let your mind expand while there are no particular thoughts. If unwanted thoughts enter your mind from time to time, acknowledge them and let them go, just as if they were a little child skipping off after getting the attention they needed. Bring your awareness back to your breath. By now you are breathing from the belly automatically and the breath has slowed down as you have settled in. Stay here for as long as you like.

Practice meditation daily and as often during the day as you need.

Toxic foods prevent us from feeling our best, and therefore our reactions to situations may not be at their best — the vicious cycle begins. Once you bring the mind and body together, the body starts to really tell you how it feels when you eat certain foods. Listen carefully. Listen. Bring your awareness into your body, and FEEL. Watch for subtle feelings and cravings as well as aversions to some things you once ate habitually. You may suddenly be satisfied with a small amount of a food you once ate large quantities of.

Now is the time to protect yourself from the continual stream of toxins entering your body via food. Have the intention to eliminate the foods that prevent you from feeling beautiful and at peace. It's time to let them go and allow your meditation practice to make it easier. Next week we will add other lifestyle adjustments regarding food and the fueling process. For now, begin to notice how your body feels as you become toxin-free.

Eliminate these
- sugar
- white flour
- caffeine
- processed and packaged foods
- milk

- diet soda
- pork
- cold cuts
- any canned or boxed food with additives

These substances accelerate aging and entropy. They are basically "dead" foods that offer no energy to your body and contribute to degeneration and decay. They prevent you from feeling the vibrance that you deserve to feel.

Be cautious with meats

- eat chicken and fish in moderation
- eat beef less often and with caution
- avoid pork
- choose organic, naturally raised meats

Our dysfunctional society accepts many "food products" that are so commonly used they are thought to be "normal." Yet, to your body when consumed, they are anything BUT normal. They set off a huge clean-up process. Transporting, filtering, and storing these toxins breaks the body down.

Notice the distinction between "common" and "normal." What are normal to the body are organic fruits and vegetables in season, fresh lean cuts of meats,

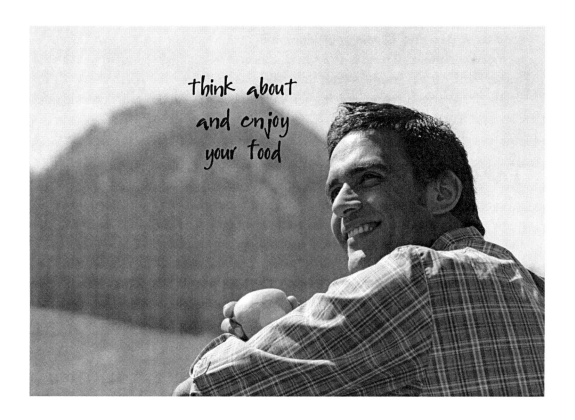

think about and enjoy your food

organically grown whole grains, and pure, clean water. Common to the "average Joe" are fast food, junk food, quick-fix meals, and pre-fabricated food products.

Anytime you open a colorful commercial package to eat what is inside, remember preservatives were added to keep it from spoiling. You ingest those preservatives right along with the food. Not only does this leave your body with less nutrition, but it also saddles the body with the huge burden of dealing with the added foreign chemicals. Many additives and preservatives are neurologically active, they alter your mood and inhibit the normal flow of body function[3].

Minimize frozen, canned, and packaged foods as much as possible. Try to stay away from leftovers and microwaved foods as well. Your body is too good for them. A rule to remember — the less time between harvesting and consumption, the more energy and intelligence the food will provide.

Food is FUEL

How you eat is how you fuel your body. This "fuel" will determine how good you feel, and feeling good is how you win the game of life. Eat when you are hungry and stop when you are satisfied. It is important to make a distinction here — this is not a diet. Dieting suggests deprivation and restriction. I think we all have had enough of that. It is OK to think about and enjoy food — really good food. Beautiful, in season produce, lean quality cuts of meat, fresh veggies seasoned and grilled. There is an endless selection of really great-tasting, satisfying "super food" that is good for your body and your mind. If you need to lose weight, it starts with eating, not restriction. You will have to eat your way thin.

Taste is Acquired

Starting from the time you were a child, the foods that were available in your home were the foods that developed your taste buds. The choice of what you ate, and how it was prepared and served, was not up to you as a child. You may have been allowed or taught to be a "picky" eater. The practice was there, and whatever mealtime meant to you was set in motion. Do Irish people like potatoes and cabbage? Do Japanese people like sushi? Do Americans like burgers and fries? Of course they do; because they were raised on it, they have a taste for it. The good news is, since taste is acquired, it is then possible to acquire a new taste over time.

---

3. Metcalfe, Dean D. Ronald Simon. "Food Allergy: Adverse Reactions to Food and Food Additives." Wiley-Blackwell, 2003 (397). August 11, 2009.

How were you taught to view food and meal times?

_____
_____
_____
_____

What was meal time like when you were a child?

_____
_____
_____
_____

Your body knows what it needs. Have you ever thought about a fresh orange or apple or a salad and had a strong desire for it, along with the feeling it would taste so good right at that moment? Unlike the driving force of a sugar craving, this is a deeper desire for the freshness, aroma, and purity of a fruit or vegetable. It is the intelligence of your body requesting specific nutrients. The intelligence of the billions of cells in your amazing body knows what it needs to function optimally. The more in tune you become with your body, the more you have the desire for fresh, clean, nutritious foods. Your body will bring you two magnificent bonuses as you meditate and become more mindful:

- You'll want MORE of the foods that your body needs to be lean, strong and feel great.
- You'll desire LESS of the foods that bring you added weight, illness and low self-esteem.

These are a small fraction of the many perks you'll receive for making food choices that may sometimes be difficult. Dieting and deprivation have no place here. Let's focus on how delicious and satisfying real, whole, fresh, super foods are. We are healing and rebuilding your body and this takes GOOD FOOD. It's time to really eat well. Continue to try a variety of produce and whole grain products. Once habitual eating is gone, it is a whole new ball game. There is a wide range of wonderful food out there that you have been missing! Foods that in the past weren't especially desirable may taste good to you now. Rather than choosing foods you have always eaten habitually in the past, keep your mind open and let your taste buds reveal to you what is really wonderful. It takes time to rid the body of the desire for hyper-taste foods, such as ranch-flavored chips, cheese-flavored crackers, or nacho-flavored "this and that." Most of these are high-sodium, genetically modified products often laced with MSG and other chemicals. Soon you will begin to actually taste food, maybe in a way you never have before — the true flavor of a grilled artichoke, a ripe avocado, fresh-squeezed orange juice, and so many other wonderful foods from nature.

Shop for organically grown foods. Your body knows just what to do with them and uses them efficiently. You can rest assured that you are not consuming unnecessary toxins along with your meals. You will be pleased at the youthful glow that starts to come over you. Listen to your body. Meditation will help you learn the language of your body. Listen. Listen.

> *Natural forces within us are the true healers of disease.*
> *— Hippocrates*

Developing Awareness

Drop a live frog into a pan of scalding hot water, and he will exert all his might to jump out of there as fast as he can. Place the same frog in a pan of warm water. Turn the heat on and slowly raise the temperature. The frog will remain in the water until he boils to death without attempting to escape. He will acclimate to the rising temperature. It is the same with our bodies' conditioning. We slowly become used to certain patterns of behavior. Just as the frog does, we acclimate and form habits that feel normal to us, even if they are destructive. As we raise our awareness, we begin to feel what is really healthy and natural for ourselves and our bodies, not what we have been conditioned to think of as "normal."

> Bob was shy as a young man. He was nervous around girls and learned to keep his hands in his pockets since it made him feel more secure. Even though he outgrew the shyness, he had a developed a stance that began with his shoulders rolling slightly forward because of the position of his hands. He got comfortable standing with his pelvis tipped slightly forward, belly protruding, causing the chest to sink inward while his hands were "hiding" in his pockets. He relied on this "stance" on many occasions — while waiting in line, shopping, or even in conversation. This long-term posturing had changed the shape of his body—he had less definition in his chest, a larger belly in front and a generally saggy, tired appearance. At first it took real intention to lift his chest up and allow his hands to be free. He added some weight training

exercises for his upper chest, back, and glutes to awaken and rebuild the areas that had atrophied.

With his own intention to release this habit and make a few small changes, Bob looks younger and stronger than he did years ago.

In her mid twenties, Diane was an energetic client of mine. One day she came to me and exclaimed, "Look at my nails! They're awful! What can I do to have nice fingernails? They're hook-shaped!" Indeed, the nails of her index finger, thumb, and middle finger were bent at a forty five-degree angle. As we chatted, the conversation soon turned to her boyfriend. She became nervous, talking at hyper-speed. I glanced down at her hands.

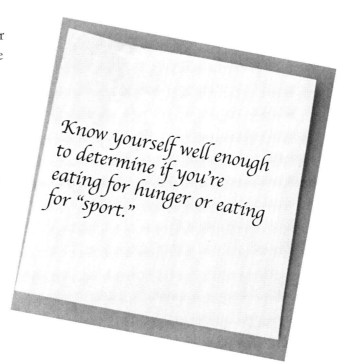

Know yourself well enough to determine if you're eating for hunger or eating for "sport."

She had placed the tip of her index finger into the pad of her thumb and was pushing, bending the nail at a 45-degree angle. Then she repeated the same thing with her middle finger as she continued to talk. As she was unaware of what she was nervously doing, I stopped her mid-sentence and said, "Diane, look down at your hands. Look at what you're doing."

It took her a moment to make the connection. Then, she gasped for breath — she was shocked. Obviously SHE was the cause of the hook-shaped nails. This had gone on for years unnoticed by Diane.

Whether it seems minor like a bent fingernail, or more obvious like changing the shape of our body, each of these incidents left the person absolutely stunned. When Bob and Diane became aware of what was happening; they both enjoyed an "I got it" moment. Once the damage was obvious, they wanted to change their behavior right away. Some ruinous behaviors are so ingrained in our routine that their familiarity can bring a false sense of comfort. We are not always aware of the effect they have on our lives. Bob may have missed out on a date or job promotion he really wanted, and Diane was confused and continually trying to hide her unsightly hands.

We are responsible for behavior that creates an unhealthy or unattractive habit. Like the frog in the warm water about to be boiled to death, we have been in the water so long we don't notice the temperature rising. Constantly furrowing the brow, sitting in a slumped position, grinding teeth, squinting the eyes, eating bites of food too big for the mouth and numerous other habits that are bad for our health and appearance could all fill this book. As we raise the awareness of our own bodies, we will let go of some things we have done habitually because they just don't feel right anymore. As we gain awareness of our own bodies, we

> **Ever wonder where your habits come from?** Your emotions and beliefs set up patterns in your life. Your stored emotions, stuck and buried, bind you to these patterns, and habits are formed like they were for Barbara, Bob, and Diane. Once you have released the stored emotions from your body, you can objectively evaluate your habits. Here's where the BONUS comes in: As they are released, your attachment to some of your bad habits and your "urge" for them are also released. If bad habits could be easily "dropped" this book would simply be a "To do" list. Habits are difficult to drop but more easily replaced. As you release your old emotional attachments, the habits connected to them serve no further purpose. Without even thinking about it, some of your old bad habits will fade away. Now is a beautiful time to replace them with the habits that nurture and rejuvenate you.

will effortlessly release habits that just don't serve a purpose anymore. This is the wisdom of your body at work.

Listen. You may begin to notice destructive behaviors and have the desire to be free of them, just as Bob and Diane did. You will gain the ability to sit quietly with yourself without fidgeting, over-thinking, or having negative thoughts pop into your mind..

Through your awareness you will find answers. Begin to observe yourself and your habits. Do you look others in the eye when engaged in conversation? Do you stand tall with your shoulders back or slump down? Do you look at the ground or straight ahead when you walk? Do you fidget with your hands or sit comfortably still? Are you a picky eater or will you try almost anything? Is your dinner table posture erect? Consider where your behaviors come from.

List here any habitual body movements that you are aware of. They may not all come to mind right now, so feel free to add them later. Leg crossing, hair flipping, slouching, jaw clenching … any and all that come to mind.
List when the behavior began.

_____
_____
_____
_____

Observe these things and more. Make notes on how you speak, walk, interact, eat, and sit. Trace back through your life, and try to find where some of these behaviors started. Prioritize some undisturbed quiet time and think back. Go over events and emotions and how they relate to some of these habits. Write about it here.

_____
_____
_____
_____
_____
_____

Understanding how these habits originate is the beginning of forming new habits that lead to health and beauty. We are laying the groundwork for the effectiveness of upcoming chapters. This may be the most challenging time of the program for you. I cannot tell you it will be easy. But I can promise you it will be worth it. Set aside at least 20 minutes of quiet time daily to ponder and journal your feelings. Be with yourself as long as you need to allow buried emotions to emerge. Feel them in your body. Make notes on where you feel discomfort in your body.

This Week's Assignments:

- Begin meditation practice daily — 20 to 30 minutes.
- Make a list of toxic foods that you need to be free of.
- Eliminate toxic foods from your list.
- Journal your feelings and experiences.

- Exercise 3 or 4 days this week at a moderate level, depending on your level of fitness. Beginners may start walking for 30–45 minutes followed by at least 5 minutes of stretching. Intermediate and advanced levels — NOW is the time to get moving! But, listen to your body and pace the intensity of your exercise. We'll add specific exercises later; for now your workouts should be 55–70 minutes followed by at least 10 minutes of stretching. Note: A great time for meditation is at the end of your workout.
- Be aware of yourself and your habits.

Continue To:

- Get rid of bad feelings and toxic emotions by going through them, letting them go.
- Review your journal and add any additional thoughts.

_____
_____
_____
_____
_____
_____
_____
_____
_____
_____
_____
_____
_____
_____
_____
_____

Today's date _____

> *Habit is habit and not to be flung
> out of the window by any man,
> but coaxed downstairs a step at a time.*
> — Mark Twain

People don't grow old. When they stop growing, they become old.

Anonymous

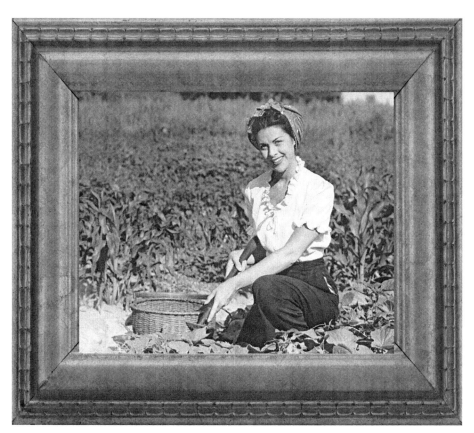

Week 3

This Week's Focus:

Face and Body Posturing
Movement and Exercise
Food Combining
The "A" List

Deborah had watched her weight all her life. She looked and felt thick through the torso; however, she was not overweight. Deborah had rounded shoulders, and her upper spine was curved, causing a "humpback." She lifted her shoulders, scrunching them upward because she thought this made her look thinner. She cared about her appearance, was always well-dressed, and maintained her hair and makeup. I wanted to understand why a health-conscious, beautifully groomed person would continue this posture. It was disfiguring her spine, and causing a sagging appearance in her neck.

As we were chatting, she told me she had developed breasts at a very young age. Her father was not happy about this, and let her know he didn't like her having a grown-up figure. She became embarrassed and didn't want the boys at school or anyone else to notice. She began to draw her chest inward, and over time this created the curve in her upper back.

This curve was lowering her ribcage, shortening her waist and thickening her midsection — she looked and felt heavier than she actually was. Then, to feel like she appeared thinner, she began drawing up or "scrunching" her shoulders. She had held this posture while walking, exercising — in all her movements since childhood. Deborah didn't notice how bad her posture was because she fixated on one thing — making sure her breasts weren't sticking out. Now she was grown and married with adult children of her own, and she no longer obsessed about her large breasts. However, she still maintained posture as if she did. At this point, in addition to a damaged spine,

> To see if rounding of the spine has begun to take over your body, try this: stand with your back against a wall with your heels touching the wall as well. Push your shoulders back until they touch, press the back of your head to the wall, lift your ribs while keeping the shoulders relaxed. Feel this position. This is not a natural stance but a good reminder of being upright. If you are straining to hold this position for a few slow breaths, you may have been inducted into the "turtle back club." This is a good way to start the day, and a nice reminder you can feel. A few moments here and you'll remember to straighten up throughout the day.

she has diminished lung capacity, headaches, varicose veins, limited mobility, and a layer of fat around her midsection — all of which had been aggravated by the posture she created because, in her own words, she wanted to look "thinner and not busty."

A properly aligned spine lifts the core up out of the pelvis, elongates the waistline, and allows it to curve inward — this presents a youthful, athletic figure. Your internal health will be enhanced because organ and nerve function are not impaired. Healing energy can flow efficiently through the channels of your body. Your lung capacity is complete and oxygenates the body efficiently. Your joints can move freely without undue strain or pressure, allowing muscles full range of motion so your body is more toned.

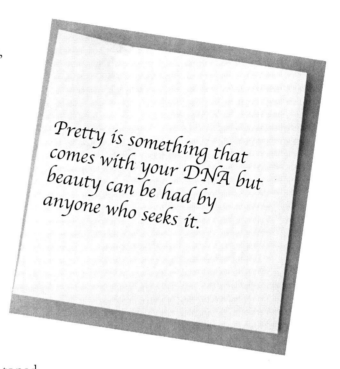

Pretty is something that comes with your DNA but beauty can be had by anyone who seeks it.

Straighten Up and Fly Right

When I was 18, I broke my leg in a parachuting accident. A few seconds after exiting the plane, I realized I was falling too fast. My chute was "breathing," or flapping in and out, because of a hole — not a good sign. My landing felt like jumping off a three-story building. I wore a cast on my lower leg for about eight weeks. When it came off, my leg was noticeably smaller. It was thin and week from atrophy. It took years to recondition my lower leg to its former size and strength.

Many of us are experiencing a similar condition in our bodies and are not even aware of it. It may not be from a marked incident such as a parachuting accident, but rather from a slow, gradual weakening of the spine due to a softened lifestyle like Deborah.

To Strengthen the Back

- Start by lying on the tummy. Lift your legs, then with arms straight out to the sides, lift them as though you are trying to bring your hands and feet up to the ceiling. Hold for 10 seconds, as if balancing on your navel. As you release back to the floor, exhale, turning to rest your cheek on the floor. Repeat three times, switching cheeks with the exhale. You'll notice improvement quickly because the muscles are there; they have simply been forgotten.

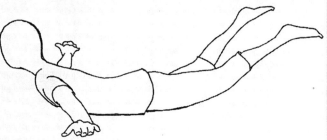

- If upper neck tension is a concern, lower arms or slightly tuck your chin until the tension is released.

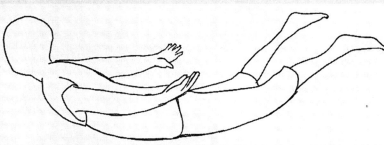

- Try extending your arms up overhead as you lengthen your hands and feet up for the advanced posture.

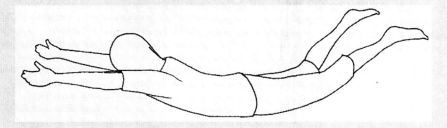

We live in a push-button world. Everyday tasks that years ago kept us moving around can today be done in a sitting position. Driving a car instead of walking, shopping online instead of cruising through the mall, pulling in for fast food instead of running in to the market and preparing dinner — the list is endless. While our lives have gotten "cushier," so have our spines. As we spend time in a sitting position, the core relaxes, the vertebrae in the spine settle, the shoulders round forward, and the stabilizer muscles weaken. The result: a torso that cannot hold itself upright, or "turtle back" posture.

So we go to the gym and exercise — we work with what we see. But it's what we can't see that could heal a weak, unstable back. An efficient workout is a balanced one, working with the front of your body AND the back. The more your back is neglected, the softer it will become. The more it is strengthened, the better your posture will be. You'll notice this as straightness in the upper back, and your clothes will hang and drape your body with a regal fit. You'll also notice your body will be upright, ribs lifted up from the pelvis, with a trimmer waistline. A spine that is aligned with a strong torso is more likely to be pain free. Back pain, weakness in the spine and weak abdominals are a package deal — if you have one, you have the other two, to some degree.

Tips for the Back

- To stretch the spine, keep a large pilates ball at home or in the office. When you are tired of sitting or feeling "soft," sit on the ball and lie back as you walk your feet out. Let the ball roll up until you can lie back with your head supported. Relax and breathe while stretched out on the ball. In a matter of moments you will be right back at your desk, only sitting up a little taller.
- When waiting in line or sitting at a desk, lift the ribs up and use the muscles around your shoulder blades to pull your shoulders back and open your chest. Let your shoulders drop down as you practice taking the top of your head up towards the ceiling, allowing the upper shoulders to stay "soft" and relaxed.
- AT ALL TIMES remember to do these things:
  - Set shoulders back and down.
  - Bring your neck and chin into the body (rather than jutting forward).
  - Lengthen upward, taking the top of your head up toward the ceiling.
  - Keep your abs tucked in and pelvis slightly tucked under.
  - If standing, spread your toes as you distribute your weight evenly between your feet.
  - Relax and breathe from your belly.
  - Watch for nervous habits such as fidgeting, shifting your weight back and forth, leaning into one hip as you stand or folding your arms while pooching your tummy forward. Release them. Switch your focus to your breath and let it calm you while you are upright, looking elegant and feeling peaceful.

The muscles that run along both sides of the backbone are stabilizers. In a properly aligned stance, your spine engages these muscles to maintain an upright posture with your chest open and shoulders back. This allows the jawline to remain lifted and less prone to sagging or a double chin. Using these stabilizers keeps them toned and strong, improving your stability and preventing your posture from "aging" with a forward slouch and protruding stomach. (You know, the little old grandma body type.) You will have the movement and walking stride of a perky, youthful person. That's a big payoff for simply standing and moving with good posture.

FACIAL POSTURE. Here's Lookin' at You, Kid.

Just as proper posturing of the spine and back muscles sculpts your physical body, proper posturing of the facial muscles sculpts and defines your face. Think of when you are tired: your body slumps forward, your back becomes rounded and your head hangs down. You may not be aware of a similar situation that is happening above your neck.

When your face is tired, it's not receiving the oxygen it needs. The delicate muscles lose tone and become more vulnerable to the pull of gravity. You become more vulnerable to drooping eyelids or jowls forming around the jaw line. When the frontal muscles of the face lose muscle tone, your upper lip drops and fewer of your front teeth are visible in your smile. Have you ever noticed that when an elderly person smiles, more of their their bottom teeth are visble than their top teeth? Nasolabial folds, the creases that run from the outside corners of your nose to the corners of your mouth, may also become more pronounced. Gravity may attempt to drag many parts of your body towards Argentina. Muscle tone is your body saying, "No thanks, I'm not going."

Catch yourself when you feel your face sag. Sit up. Lift your face up and breathe. Find a neutral position that is not as exaggerated as the exercise, and wear it in your face as often as possible. Not a surprised expression, it's rather a feeling of "awakeness." Avoid resting your elbows on a table with your face in your hands — it weakens the back and wrinkles the face and can become a habit. Use your spine and back to sit up. Keep your hands away from your face. Resist the urge to rub your eyes. This spreads germs and intensifies wrinkles by stretching the skin. Awareness of your facial posturing will provide a smoother, less wrinkled and fresher face.

The lines and wrinkles in your face are there because emotion, stress, imbalanced diet or other circumstances in your life have put them there[1]. You

---

1. Chopra, Deepak. Ageless Body Timeless Mind. New York: Harmony Books, 1993.

have the power to release lines from your face. It doesn't take an injection to stop wrinkling your face. You can do it simply and more beautifully with intention.

Paralyzing an area of your face to avoid wrinkles is the same school of thought as wiring your jaw shut because you need to lose a few pounds. To give up the warmth or sweet expression you have when you smile or feel compassion for a frozen, desolate face with fewer wrinkles is not a good trade off. Through your awareness, it is possible to reduce the lines and wrinkles in your face. With these exercises, a super-foods eating plan, oxygen and intention, you have the ability to create your own fresh and ageless look. It's like going back in time only better, because of the wisdom you're gaining and the person you're becoming.

Try this exercise to tone the facial muscles. A great time for this is just after applying your moisturizer:

> Take your awareness to your face. Lift upward and out on all the muscles you can feel in your forehead as if you were gently surprised, but without moving your eyelids or straining to raise your eyebrows. These are called the occipito frontalis muscles; the temporalis muscles are to the sides and above your ears. Keep your eyelids neutral. Take a few deep breaths, hold here for a few seconds and then release. Now focus on the frontal muscles of your face. Keep your lips together and, without wrinkling your upper lip, gently press your lips together as you lift up on the muscles that run across your cheek bones. Pull outward with the corners of your mouth as if pursing your lips while keeping them smooth — no wrinkles. Do not squint your eyes. Take a few deep breaths as you hold this posture. Gently pat for a few seconds all over the face to stimulate collagen and improve circulation.
> Repeat daily.

Don't jump out of an airplane with a hole in your parachute. Straighten up and you'll FLY RIGHT.

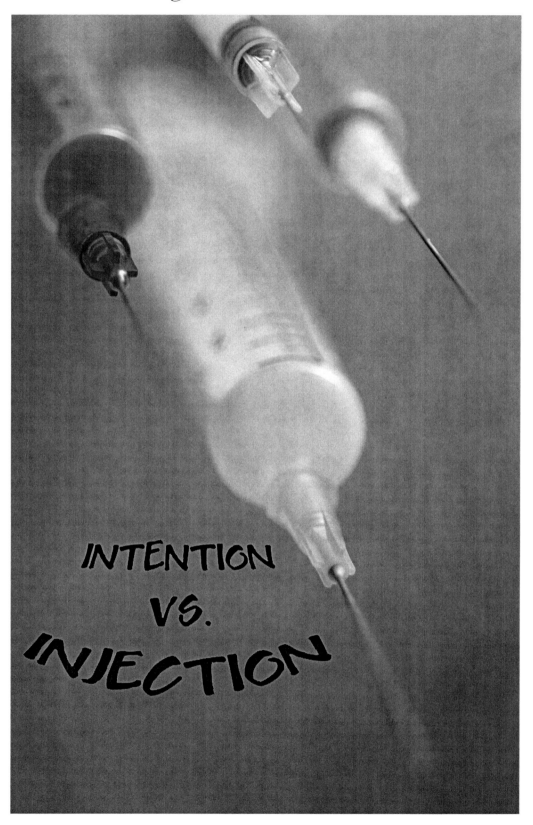

INTENTION VS. INJECTION

INJECTION

Pros
- It's fast.
- You don't have to take responsibility for your face; you hand over that responsibility to the person who is giving you the injection.

Cons
- A paralyzed face is lifeless and void of pleasant calmness.
- Paralyzing facial tissues creates atrophy, which can cause sagging.
- There is a risk of mistreatment: the wrong muscles may be paralyzed, causing a drooping eye, brow, or other disfigurement.
- It can be painful, and expensive.
- Treatments must be redone every few months.
- Scheduling appointments and waiting in the doctor's office is time consuming.

INTENTION

Pros
- Better way to relieve stress and headaches.
- It gets easier the more you practice.
- The effects are lifelong.
- The skin has a natural glow.
- It's free.
- You feel more calm as you release the tension in the face.
- Your smile is still your own.
- You maintain your youthful, recognizable face.
- Your face can authentically display sweetness, warmth, and affection.

Cons
- It takes practice to make it a habit.
- The results are not immediate; instead, they come over time.

Walking

When you are awake you are in perpetual motion. Walking is the universal mode of movement. The average person walks approximately two to three miles every day, depending on their level of activity[2]. It takes about 2,000 steps to equal one mile, so that means the average person walks about 6,000 steps every day.

Since walking is the basic movement of life, it is crucial that it be efficient and not tax the body in any way. Our posture should protect our joints at all times. Walking with absolute correctness can prevent damage to our joints, enable correct breath work, tone the torso, and — last but not least — carry us through the situations of life with grace and elegance. So often we take walking for granted, giving it no thought or conscious effort when, in fact, there are many rewards we can reap by adjusting our walking and movement posture.

Think of all the time in your life that is spent getting from place to place. Walking should be brisk and deliberate. Walking for exercise is a perfect opportunity to clear your mind, feel peaceful, and focus on your inner self. Avoid walking paths that have garbage cans, speeding traffic, barking dogs, or any other unpleasant or stressful situations. Your walking path should have beauty and fresh air if possible. A quiet neighborhood or outdoor track is a great place to free your mind because fewer distractions mean less stress.

Feel Like Dancing?

We were sitting around at a family reunion when two little nieces, about four and six years old, burst into a dance. With no music playing, there was twirling, free-styling, and assorted "fly girl" moves. It was unplanned; they just felt it and went with it as if the open space of the gymnasium floor had called to them. With laughter between his words my dad said, "Wouldn't it be great to feel that good — so good you just wanted to dance!" I wondered why some of us grown-ups don't feel that way.

A personal training student of mine announced before a workout that she was "allergic" to exercise, hates doing it, and isn't good at it. She was forcing herself to get in shape for a class reunion and, after a couple of sessions, she told me about the time in her seventh grade gym class she came in last in the mile run, and all the kids stood there waiting for her to cross the finish line. Then there was the getting picked last for dodge ball and never being able to do the splits like her friends. A lot of beliefs were

---

2. "How Many Steps Do You Walk Each Day?" The Walking Site, 2005. August 19, 2009

tied up in those memories. She believed she just wasn't good at any kind of movement and associated exercise with failure and shame. However, before she learned to be ashamed of her body's performance, at some point she felt like my two little nieces on the gym floor.

Anyone raising a toddler can tell you it's an all-day chasing game. We start out active, we do cartwheels on the lawn, and we run and play until someone tells us we're not good at it. Then we find other things to do, and in this age of technology there are plenty of other sedentary things to do. Whether or not you like to exercise, your body rejoices in movement. By understanding yourself and your feelings about exercise, you'll be able to release any negative feelings about movement.

Describe your level of activity as a child:
_____
_____

How did gym class attendance as a child make you feel?
_____
_____

As a teenager?
_____
_____

Were you ever teased because of your physical size or ability to perform in sports and activities?
_____

What games or sports were you praised for doing well?
_____

Were you ever punished with exercise, i.e., made to run an extra lap because you messed up in the game?
_____

Was your family an active or sedentary bunch? Did they enjoy outdoor sports or indoor technology? Describe the individuals you were raised around.
_____
_____

Somewhere in our memory banks are positive memories of our bodies moving freely and joyously. If we can access our fond memories of that constantly-in-motion inner kid, we can begin to view our exercise time as a treat. Celebrate the gift and blessing it is to have an amazing healing machine that moves. Have compassion for yourself if you can't quite hit that new yoga pose, be thrilled about that extra half mile you added to your morning walk, or smile as you enter your fitness club. But, be ready to burst into dance and if you begin to feel those freestyle moves coming on, I hope you go with it!

When Walking, Remember To

- Lift your ribs to bring the core up out of your pelvis.
- Relax the shoulders. Set them back and down.
- Allow the natural swing of your arms to propel you forward.
- Keep the chin tucked slightly. Make sure the neck is in line, not jutting forward.
- Take the top of your head straight up, lifting up towards the sky.
- Let go of any swinging, swaying, or excess movement.
- Glide.
- Aim your toes straight ahead of your heels, facing ahead rather than turned out or inward.
- Step forward, heel first. Roll forward through the balls of the feet, then through the toes.
- Breathe from the abdomen.
- Look ahead, not down at the ground. Your peripheral vision will help you travel carefully, allowing you to stay upright, feel elegant, and enjoy the beauty of your surroundings.

Exercise

When I was a young single mother with very little time or money, I would go to a nearby park. There was a large section of the park where I could walk the circumference. I would take my two little boys and put them in the center where I could see them every step of the way. We brought wheel toys, kites, and bubbles. I would walk or jog the circumference of the park around them while they played and waved at me. If they needed me they could run to me, and it was a safe place. At first they weren't sure they wanted me to go that far away, but we figured out a system so that everyone had a good time and got some fresh air. I would finish in the center with them, stretching in the grass. Core work would follow as I listened to what they had been doing. It was a wonderful workout at a time in my life when there seemed to be no other way. Even now I still have memories of them waving to me while playing in that park.

You don't need the perfect scenario in order to have time to exercise. There are many options. No matter what phase of life you are in or what your daily schedule is like, all areas of life improve with exercise. It brings oxygen needed for clear thought, smooth skin, healing, improved organ function, blood production, muscle and bone development and enhanced body function all around. Exercise is your time to regroup and use your body, which is more important than just burning calories. If your goal is strictly to burn calories, you are perceiving your body as a machine. You are an intelligent, organic, miraculous being made of energy. Exercise is much more than calorie burning. It's your play time, a chance to bring your mind and body together. It brings needed oxygen to all the cells of your body, slowing down the aging process. It simultaneously relieves stress and tones your body.

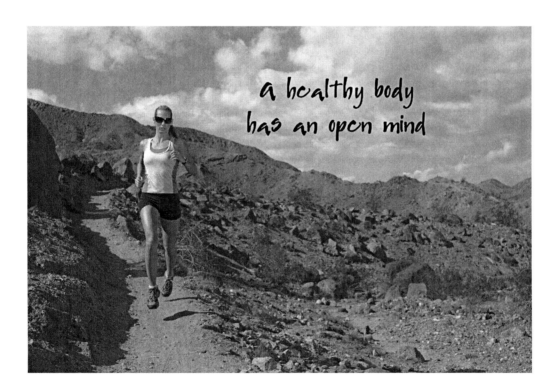

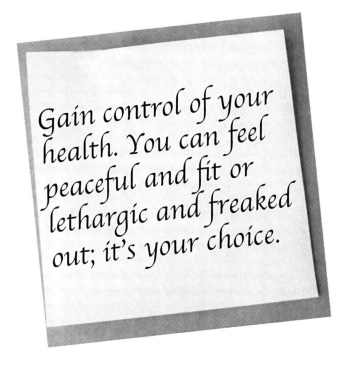

Gain control of your health. You can feel peaceful and fit or lethargic and freaked out; it's your choice.

I have developed a mind and body sculpting workout that resculpts the shape of the body while releasing stored emotion and stress. Various modalities and transitions cause this class to be the most efficient, effective, age-reversing program that I have encountered. If you do not have access to the DVD or live class, you can create a workout and personalize it according to your lifestyle and personal preferences. As you move through this program, we will gradually add in some of the postures and exercises.

Whether you choose the controlled setting of the gym or fresh air outdoors, find movement that you enjoy and apply it to your daily life so that it takes precedence over anything else. If this time for exercise is set aside as a priority then scheduling conflicts will disappear. You can plan your life around this time knowing that whatever other activities fill the day, you feel great and have energy because you have had "your" time and are ready and willing to face any challenge.

I have friends whose teenage children attend a 6 a.m. religion class before school. Since these moms and dads are up to drop the kids off, they walk together for that hour and return to the church in time to pick the kids up. This may not have been their first choice of exercise scenarios, but they found a way to bring an exercise routine into their busy lives. Once they acclimated to the earlier workout schedule, they loved it because they were finished early and could get on with their day. Even with time constraints and a difficult situation, they made it work.

There are many demands on our time and attention. We get so busy "doing" and "going" and "achieving" that priorities continually get reshuffled. Once exercise is a part of your life, there will be no more having to decide, "Should I work out this morning or not?" You have already committed to it, and it is simply part of your day. It is wonderful to be free of always having to MAKE THE CHOICE. Just go, even if it feels mechanical at first. Walk yourself through it because soon your body will crave it. Your lean, strong, energetic body and clear mind are only the beginning of the rewards.

As your personal trainer, I would put together a circuit or group of exercises that focus on the areas that need improvement while protecting any former injuries or weaknesses. I would design a workout that takes in your personal preferences such as being indoors or out, being with a group or alone, the type of music to add, and so forth. But you can make these choices for yourself and I'll include some basic guidelines here for you. Whatever you choose for exercise, it should include these things:

1. Before you start, take a moment to begin every workout with a few meditative breaths, focusing on appreciation for your body and what a gift it is to be able to move and use your body. Clear your mind as you warm up with five minutes of gentle stretching.

2. Align your spine, keeping the chest open and neck carriage tucked in. Avoid slouching as you begin walking, jogging, running, or other form of cardio.

3. Do at least 20–25 minutes of cardio — vigorous exercise that will elevate your heart rate such as brisk walking with intermittent jogging, or uphill climbing .

4. Exercise your abdominals with varied crunches and leg lifts at least 10 minutes to tone the core and back.

5. End the active part of your workout with 15 minutes of deep stretching to tone your body.

6. Finish with a few minutes of meditation in a quiet place. Close your eyes, erase your thoughts, and just breathe. Take your time getting up when you're ready.

I will make more exercise recommendations later, but for this week you should exercise three to four times. Concentrate on the blessing of being in control of the movement of your body and what a gift it is to you.

Journal how you feel about your body and exercise.

_____
_____
_____

How would you like to feel about your body and exercise?

_____
_____

Track your exercise days and time for this week on your chart in the back of your manual.

Food Combining

Do you remember going to the pharmacy when you were a little kid? I do. I would meander through the store looking around at the beauty and health products and wonder which ones did what. I remember the small section for stomach aids. There were several things: pink stuff for indigestion and other stuff for diarrhea. When you walk into any pharmacy today, brace yourself — you'll likely find several very long aisles full of every kind of medication for digestion you can imagine. Pills for bloating, pills for gas, liquid elixirs for both, something for acid reflux, capsules for constipation, pills to help you digest certain foods after you have eaten them — so many it boggles the mind!

Stomach and digestive problems are created by diet and are at an all time high. We "need" these various treatments because of what and how we eat. We've programmed our taste buds to enjoy modified and denatured foods loaded with flavor enhancers. Quick meals, prepared and eaten in a hurry, may taste good but require an arsenal of the above-mentioned pills or formulas to manage the discomfort they bring. That discomfort is your body saying, "Please help me out here."

> Have the intention to feel vital, move freely, and have a more graceful countenance from this moment on.

Foods have become faster and easier to prepare, which means they have been processed or partially cooked with their natural value stripped away. There are thousands of toxic chemical additives that preserve odor and color, even though the food value has diminished[3]. A typical so-called "balanced meal" might be a plate full of artificial foods that should not be eaten together. The average American diet brings the average American stomach

---

3. "Toxic Food Additives." Idea Connection. 2007–2009. Online Data Services Ltd. 19 June 2009. www.ideaconnection.com/solutions/6488-toxic-food-additives.html

troubles. Walking through your local pharmacy illustrates that these troubles are many. More and more products will continue to enter the market to help your body cope with the ravages of artificial foods eaten in bad combinations.

> Detoxification is often thought of as needed after an extended period of careless eating and drinking. Or when feeling so tired and lethargic that "it's time to do something." But the fact is, your body is in the continual process of purifying itself naturally. Sweating, exhaling, and eliminating are some of the ways your physical wastes are processed every day. Detoxifaction should not be harsh nor extreme. Ultimately you are detoxifying every system of your body with each good choice you make. The goal is to live a lifestyle that allows your body to be purified, ageless, and disease-free. Watch for clearer skin, a flatter tummy, ease of digestion, a peaceful feeling inside, and increased ability to focus. Watch your face and body closely and be sure to journal about every positive change you notice and the date you notice it.

Not Just What, but When

Eliminating toxic foods is the first step towards gaining control of your health and beauty. Finding wellness takes more than simply not eating unhealthy foods. Let's focus on how to eat so there is the maximum energy available to you, so your metabolism is working at its optimum rate, so excess pounds drop away effortlessly and your tummy is flat, so you feel better than you ever have. You won't walk down the stomach-aid section of the pharmacy ever again, either! It is not only possible, it will happen if you understand the concepts of food combining and empower yourself to implement them into your life. Allowing digestion to operate optimally brings longevity, energy, and a flat tummy[4].

Seasons and Cycles

Mother Nature operates in cycles. Man has aligned himself with these cycles for centuries. Fruit trees need a season to grow and a season to ripen. Fruit is gathered

---

4. Moss Green. "How to Detoxify Your Body Naturally." The Voice of Women 2009. 18 August 2009. www.bellaonline.com/articles/art7703.asp.

when it is plentiful and then when it is gone it needs time before the tree can blossom again. Throughout history, these cycles have been honored. When it was time for the corn harvest, corn was plentiful. Meat was hunted and plentiful for a time and then unavailable when snow covered the ground. These cycles naturally brought food combining to man through the ages, and there wasn't a pharmacy in sight to go get the "pink stuff" for your stomach.

> *If anything is sacred, the human body is sacred.*
> — Walt Whitman

In 1941, the National Nutrition Conference came up with the Recommended Dietary Allowance (RDA) for Americans to follow[5]. A food pyramid was created and we all started eating a whole plate full of foods together — a so-called "balanced" diet. Engineers figured out how to bleach whole wheat and then enrich it again, making bread lighter and softer. We learned to freeze, dehydrate, reconstitute, pre-mix, pre-bake, and prefabricate breakfast, lunch, dinner and snack foods. It all seemed so modern and high-tech and everyone jumped on the band wagon. As these developments increased, the health of this country declined.

"Loa's" Super Food Combining

The principles of food combining are dictated by digestive chemistry. Foods are not all digested the same way. Let's work WITH the science of your body[6].

- Starchy foods require an alkaline digestive medium, which is supplied initially in the mouth by the enzyme ptyalin.
- Protein foods require an acid medium for digestion — hydrochloric acid.
- As you may remember from chemistry class, acids and bases (alkalis) neutralize each other. If you eat a starch with a protein, digestion is impaired or completely arrested. Anytime two or more foods are eaten at the same time, and those foods require opposite conditions for digestion, the digestive process struggles and slows down. Bacteria ferments and decomposes undigested food. The undigested food mass can cause various kinds of digestive disorders, giving off poisonous by-products that inhibit nerve function and the body's ability to heal itself. And yet your amazing body plugs along, doing the best it can.

---

5. ALLGOV, Center for Nutrition Policy and Promotion. "Everything our Government Really Does." 12 June 2009. www.allgov.com/agency/center-for-nutrition-policy-and-promotion.
6. Marci, Kat. "Healthy Food Combining." 20 January 2009. www.fitconnect.com/fitness-communities/healthy-food-combining-85.

Correct food combinations are important, not only for digestion but utilization and assimilation of the nutrients in all foods. Enzyme breakdown happens naturally, while bacterial breakdown is quite destructive. Bacterial breakdown creates toxic gases which manifest in the body as bloating, burping, flatulence, candida, fatigue, headaches, constipation, diarrhea, low back pain, and so on. This serves as a reminder that all illness and aging starts in the bowel[7]. However, your digestive tract can be your highway to beauty and remaining ageless. But if you eat like the average American, it can lead to pain and suffering. The good news is you get to decide which you'd rather have. The principles of super food combining may seem confusing at first, but once you've understood them and felt the effects in your body, you'll never want to eat any other way. And you'll NEVER have to ask diet questions such as, "Am I getting enough fiber and protein?" "Are there too many carbs in this?" "Is this fattening?" "Does this have too many calories?" Those concerns are all gone because nature has taken care of that in the organic design of whole foods, plus you are eating them in combinations that allow digestion to work efficiently. Eating can be stress-free and empowering.

Freedom from all those diet-worries is liberating. Now instead you might ask; "What will this do for my body?" "Will this make me feel energetic or sluggish?" "Am I eating in proper combination so I can digest this without consequences?"

Food combining works with your body naturally. You have salivary glands in your lips, cheeks, tongue, and mouth that release enzymes and electrolytes to begin the breakdown process. Miraculously, your body sends what is needed. Proteins and carbohydrates digest at different rates and require different enzymes and environments for digestion. If these various enzymes are delivered to the stomach at the same time, they render each other ineffective or cancel each other out. This brings the digestion process to a halt. More energy is required of your body to get things sorted out and back on track. Your system bogs down. Spending this energy unnecessarily leaves you feeling tired and less vital, as well as suffering from bloating, gas and a worn-out stomach. The key is eating real, organic, unprocessed foods at the right times in the proper combinations.

Fruits

Fruits digest faster than any other foods and should be eaten alone. If they are eaten at the end of a meal, your body will release the enzymes needed for their digestion into an already full stomach. As the fruit digests and moves past the undigested proteins and carbs it causes gas and discomfort. The concept of food combining has been around for many years. Did your grandmother ever say to you, "Don't eat watermelon after your dinner"? She was absolutely right.

---

7. Wright, Theresa. "Illness." Nuconcepts. 18 August 2009. www.nuconceptsinc.com/illness.htm.

Carbs

Carbohydrates (sugars and starches) are a fuel source to your body. When eaten, carbohydrates break down into glucose, which causes your glycemic index (or blood sugar level) to rise. When blood sugar is elevated, the pancreas secretes the hormone insulin. Insulin is the hormone that tries to balance the level of blood sugar by carrying the excess glucose to the cells where it will be burned for energy[8]. When the sugar is stored safely in the cells, the level of your blood sugar is balanced. If your cells have all the sugar they can handle and cannot accept any more, then the insulin will send the extra sugar to be stored as fat, keeping it on hand for later use (and, you guessed it, you gain weight).

Rather than simple sugars, the carbs in your diet should be complex carbs, such as veggies and whole-grain products. As we said in the last chapter, simple (refined, processed) carbohydrates such as sugar, white rice, white bread, and any other products that contain white flour need to be eliminated from the diet. Potatoes are a whole food but should be avoided while trying to lose weight. Simple carbs "spike" the blood sugar, or cause it to elevate too quickly. Ever felt a sugar rush? This is caused by having too much insulin in the bloodstream. And since your body is so wonderfully efficient, if there is more insulin in the blood than the body needs, the unused carbs are stored as fat.

As you can see, it is essential to be in tune with your body, to recognize how you feel when your body is secreting excess insulin and to know which foods are responsible. Know your body and be aware of how sugar makes you feel. Be aware of headaches, dizziness, crankiness, and fatigue. All can come from the crash after a sugar high. Recognize these symptoms and equate them to sugar consumption. Let your body and mind awareness guide your food choices.

Let's Keep It Real

There's no upside to sugar consumption. Consuming sugar is like hitting your thumb with a hammer. You may smack it lightly by having just a bite, or you may smash it until it's a bloody stump by bingeing. With every smack of the hammer your body will have to work to repair the damage, even though you can't see it. It is up to you to decide when to stop swinging the hammer. You are the proprietor of this body, so learning to regulate your insulin levels is up to you. When insulin levels are regulated, your weight and hormones will be regulated as well.

When your body needs energy, it looks first for carbs to burn as fuel. If there aren't enough stored carbohydrates available, your body will start to use the fat

---

8. Norman, James, M.D. "Diabetes: What is Insulin?" Endocrineweb, Vertical Health. 18 August 2009. www.endocrineweb.com/diabetes/2insulin.html.

reserves. Because you are limiting sugars and starches, your body will become more efficient at locating and burning fat. Hormones will stay in balance and along with hormone balance comes a sense of peace, clarity of thought, less wrinkling of the skin, longevity and decreased risk for cancer and other diseases, plus one of my favorite bonuses — the glow or vitality that comes to your face. Food combining and eliminating sugar helps to keep hormones balanced and is the most powerful, age-defying beauty treatment of all.

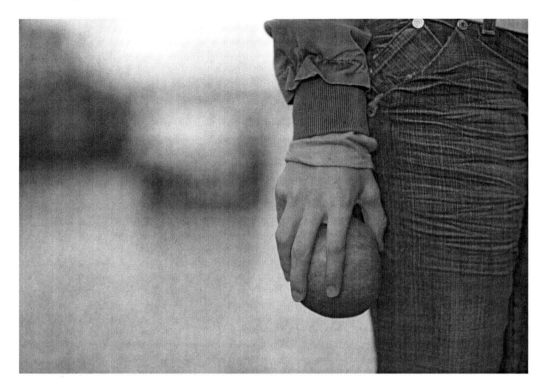

In your quest for health, remember, your hormones are the **BIG KAHUNA, the head honcho, the boss, the main thing**. When hormone levels are in check, the other systems of your body are free to function more efficiently, and the energy of your body will flow.

Since you have eliminated the toxic foods that were listed in the previous chapter, you will already be feeling and looking better. There is no place in your life for the stress that comes from being on a restricted diet. These guidelines are a lifestyle, and if I had to name it, I'd call it **IF GOD MADE IT** plan. If it is a natural, wholesome food from nature, not only is it welcome, but it will bring you health, nutrition, and vitality. If it is man-made, processed, packaged, or altered in some way, then it is not for your body. Eating the right foods in the proper combination will bring you a lean, healthy body, and all the while you will be satisfied because you are enjoying really great food. Having a love for good food will help you with this part of the program.

I came to appreciate the value of the "A" List through 30-plus years of doing makeup for "A" List actors in the film and television industry. Just as Hollywood assigns its most powerful, desirable actors to the "A" List, your "A" List also assigns power and desirability to the super foods your body deserves.

These super antioxidants are necessary to heal and balance your systems. The goal here is to have as many different "A" List items as you can each day. (Notice I didn't say "as much of" as you can.) I don't like to list quantities, but on the "A" List I need to. **(U)** means unlimited, have as much as you like. It's better to move around the list than have too much of one item.

By combining your foods correctly and incorporating more of the "A" List foods, you will be on your way to a healthy and renewed body. All the energy being trapped in your digestive system, trying to sort out what enzymes to send in, will now be freed up to heal and renew your body. You will feel more energy while losing unwanted pounds that are hanging on to your body. Digestive problems, stomach acid, bloating and gas will fall by the wayside. Once you have tried it

The "A" List

- Mangosteen, acai, or pomegranate juice, 3 oz.
- Detox, white, green, or ginger tea, 1 cup
- Wheat grass-start with single shots (1 oz.), work up to double (2 oz.)
- Blueberries, goji berries, or fresh pineapple chunks, large handful or about ½ cup
- Grapefruit, half or 1 whole
- Red pepper (U)
- Almonds — raw and unblanched, small handful
- Garlic (U)
- Onions (U)
- Flax seed (U)
- Sprouts, micro greens, or chopped wheat grass (U)
- Fresh squeezed vegetable juice, such as carrot-beet-ginger-parsley (or your favorite combination), 8 to 12 oz.
- Kale, spinach (U)
- Beets and sweet potatoes, about ½ cup

**Check with your doctor regarding any medications you are taking, especially before eating grapefruit. .
**Avoid ginger tea if you're experiencing menopausal hot flashes.

and seen and felt how natural eating is better to the body, you will never want to eat any other way. You will become so lean you will never think about dieting again, and your body will heal and rebuild itself rather than being overloaded with digestive problems that deplete your energy, break down the body's filter system, and expedite the aging process.

The "A" List — DEFINED

These are power foods; they build and heal the body. Try to incorporate them into your day in different ways and as often as you can. You can find most of these in your local market in the organic section or specialty grocery stores like Whole Foods.

Wheat grass is loaded with chlorophyll and acts as a powerful anti-inflammatory agent. It helps form healthy blood cells, has an antibacterial effect, and speeds up healing. Glowing, smooth skin is a favorite benefit of wheat grass juice. This inexpensive super nutritious food into ounces or "shots." Begin by having a one ounce shot on two occasions anytime during the week. Work up to three shots per week. Find out the quick access route to juice spots near your frequently traveled paths. You'll soon know the most convenient route and best time of day to stop in.

Flax seed is considered a modern miracle food because of its high alpha linolenic acid (Omega 3 fatty acid) content. It lowers cholesterol and blood pressure and reduces the risk of heart attack by preventing platelets from becoming "sticky." It's also rich in the disease-fighting agent lignan. It adds a nutty flavor and crunch and can be sprinkled on most any dish: toast, a salad, blended in a smoothie — the sky is the limit. Use your sugar bowl (maybe even a pretty vintage one) to store flax seed in the fridge; the little spoon is handy as well.

Pineapple contains Bromelain, a natural anti-inflammatory that encourages healing, reduces pain, and has many other health benefits. It can help relieve rheumatoid arthritis symptoms and promote good digestion. Pineapples also provide an ample supply of vitamin C — a commonly known antioxidant that protects the body from free radical damage, boosts the immune system, metabolizes cholesterol, and builds healthy collagen (there's the glowing, smooth skin starting to happen!). Pineapple is a powerful healer to the body. Cut off the top, slice in half length-wise, cover one side, and store in the refrigerator. Use a sharp knife to remove skin and cut into bite-size cubes. Keep in an airtight container in the refrigerator for easy access. Have it first thing in the morning.

Pomegranates are extremely rich in polyphenolic compounds. They have anti-tumor and cancer-fighting properties. A powerful antioxidant, this seedy fruit fights heart disease by preventing fatty deposits from collecting on arterial walls. Use them in unexpected places like green salads, salsa, sauces, and garnishes.

Blueberries lower your risk of cancer and heart disease and are anti-inflammatory. Since inflammation is the main driving force of any chronic disease, they're a great "power tool" for your body. Eat about a half-cup daily. When you can't find them fresh, eat them frozen. They are also packed with phytoflavonoids and are high in potassium and vitamin C. The darker in color they are, the higher the antioxidant potential.

Goji berries are sometimes called Wolfberries, and are some of the most nutrient dense fruits on the planet. They contain 18 kinds of amino acids (right up there with bee pollen), including all 8 essential amino acids and up to 21 trace minerals. Loaded with B vitamins and iron, their polysaccharides strengthen the immune system and are known for anti-aging properties. Look for them in health-conscious grocery stores.

Acai berries are loaded with anthocyanins, or strong antioxidants, to heal the body. They contain almost ideal protein "building blocks" in their essential amino acid complex. They have it all — omega fatty acids, calcium, fiber, and vitamins. You may have to get this power food in juice form (the pulp is juiced with it), as it comes from South America.

- Note: Goji and Acai berries were not on the "A" List because they are exotic and transported here in various ways and sometimes difficult to find. Whether frozen, dried, or however you find them, they are definitely "A" List-worthy and should be used in small amounts.
- Mangosteen juice contains xanthones, which help to wipe out the free radicals racing around inside trying to age us. It has anti-inflammatory properties, which help with joint pain, arthritis, and premature aging. Loaded with nutrients and healing properties, it comes from Southeast Asia, so it may also have to be used in juice form.
- Note: Goji, Acai, and Mangosteen grow primarily in other corners of the world so use caution when purchasing. They may be frozen or juiced but, given their nutritional value, they're definitely on the "A" List. Make sure there is no added sugar, preservatives, or water. When you look at the price, consider what you are getting — they're worth it! When taken in juice form, small servings are suggested.

Almonds will keep hunger and cravings at bay. Because of the way they are absorbed into the body, they improve satiety. High in protein and flavenoids, they are the most nutritionally packed of nuts, and they lower cholesterol and regulate blood sugar. They are essential for balancing your hormones, one of our main objectives. Because of high levels of magnesium and potassium, they improve blood flow, carrying nutrients and oxygen to the body. Make them a habit. Separate a bag of raw almonds into single serving-size bags (about an ounce or handful) and keep in your freezer for quick access. Keep a bag in your car and one at your desk. Make this power snack part of your day — almonds are a must-have.

Micro greens add a wonderful crunch to any vegetable sandwich. They are packed with antioxidant properties. Throw them in salads, on soups, in sandwiches — anywhere you like. They are a designer food and currently very popular in fine restaurants because they're so versatile. They are tasty when seasoned with fresh cracked lemon pepper. Alternate with sprouts of your choice. (Broccoli sprouts have 50 times the amount of sulforaphane by weight as mature broccoli.) Look for them near the lettuce and herbs section.

Sweet Potatoes are loaded with carotenoids, vitamin C, calcium, iron, potassium, and fiber. This complex carbohydrate is a nutritional hard-hitter that builds beautiful skin. Line the bottom of your oven and bake them slowly. Mash with freshly cracked sea salt and pepper and a few drops of agave nectar. Kids like them too.

> *Health is worth more than learning.*
> *— Thomas Jefferson*

Spinach and Kale are full of protein, fiber, calcium, potassium, niacin, and zinc, and plenty of vitamins and anti-inflammatory properties. They taste great when flavored with garlic and onions, and they cook down so the nutritional punch is multiplied. Loaded with anti-inflammatory properties, plus they are reasonably priced.

Beets contain betacyanin, a pigment that gives them their beautiful red color, and has powerful cancer-fighting properties. Beets increase antioxidant enzymes in the liver that protect liver cells from free radical damage. They contain powerful nutrient compounds that help guard against birth defects, heart disease, and certain cancers.

The "Allium Family" takes in shallots, onions, scallions, chives, leeks, and garlic. All assist the liver in detoxifying the body by getting rid of toxins and carcinogens. Garlic is a natural antibiotic and disease-fighter. It lowers blood lipid levels and helps to stabilize blood sugar levels. It's easy to cook with, so use it whenever possible.

Food Combining

Combining your food correctly takes thought at first, but it becomes very simple and second nature because it is natural to your body. Food is meant to be enjoyed. Learn to appreciate really good produce — a crisp, sweet apple, a perfectly ripened avocado, a fresh, good quality cut of meat, or a ruby-red grapefruit picked in season. To have a passion for truly great food is wonderful. Living life deprived, restricted, or on a diet stifles your spirit. Guilt has no place in your life. Once you truly appreciate good food and have committed to keep the junk (packaged, processed, sugared, or fake) food out of your body, your internal struggle with food will be gone. That's when it gets really fun. You eat what you want and want what you eat! Listen to your body. If you really listen, it will tell you which foods you need. The intelligence of your body is the best guide to health and beauty. Be aware of the lean, light feeling you have as you lose weight. Embrace that feeling and hold it in your body memory.

Food Combining Guidelines

1. All foods should be organic. Eat organically grown foods that are fresh, not frozen or reheated. Eat produce as close to harvest as possible. "Pick and eat" whenever you can.

2. Fruit should always be eaten alone. Melons should not be combined with other fruits ("eat 'em alone or leave 'em alone"). Your body works in cycles and needs high water-content foods, especially in the morning. Make sure you have fruit before noon. After eating fruit, wait at least 20 minutes before eating a carb or 2 hours before eating a protein.
   - Never eat fruit at the end of a meal.
   - Lettuce and celery can combine with fruit such as apples or pears.

Note: For sensitive stomachs or existing digestive disorders, you may want to also keep types of fruit separated. Combine fruits according to their type: "sweet," "acid," "melon," or "citrus." Sweet fruits = bananas, mangos, papayas, dried fruits, persimmons, and prunes. Acid fruits = all others except citrus and melons.

3. Eat proteins, vegetables, and fats together, but NOT with carbs: Do not combine meat with bread or other starches. Eat only one kind of lean meat at a meal. Eat salmon 2–3 times per week. Avoid pork, and eat beef in moderation.

4. Carbs can be eaten with vegetables but not with fats. All carbs should be whole grain. Add quinoa, spelt, barley, and other grains. Corn, peas, potatoes, pumpkins, yams, and carrots are starches. Combine them as though they were carbs.

5. Do not drink while you eat. Drink at least 20 minutes before a meal or wait until your stomach has handled the meal, about an hour after you have eaten. Never "wash food down."

6. Keep mealtime separate from stress, rushing, bad feelings, or anxiousness. Take the time to sit down, relax with your family or friends, and enjoy the food. Avoid multi-tasking, such as driving or watching TV while eating.

7. Absolutely NO preservatives or processed foods. They are garbage to you. Soon your hormones will balance, and cravings for these will go away. Your body is too good for them. Avoid these like the plague — they ARE the plague:
   - white flour; white rice; sugar; bottled dressings or sauces; soda; margarine; fast food; anything out of a package, bag, tub, box, or wrapper; anything pre-made, processed past its prime or stale; natural and artificial flavorings, MSG, BHT, nitrates; and anything you can't pronounce.

8. Do not skip meals. Be present when eating and stop when satisfied. Be aware of how awful you feel when you are full. Chew your food to liquid consistency. As you become more aware of your body through the meditation process, you will have less desire to overeat. If you feel like eating light, do so. Avoid foods that make you feel full and heavy.

9. Use fresh herbs, garlic, and onions liberally to season food.

10. Red meat and fried foods should be eaten sparingly. Coconut is a starch, protein, and saturated fat combination — avoid it while training.

Let's Drop The "D" Bomb

List here diets you have tried in the past.
_____
_____
_____
_____
_____

In trying to lose weight, what circumstances have helped you to feel successful?
_____
_____
_____
_____
_____

Diets are depressing because in the long run, they don't work. Dieting means counting calories, wondering if you had one bite too many, and feeling guilty, deprived, and restricted. It means going to battle with the science of your body. And if you want to go head to head with science, let me tell you right now, you cannot beat it. Dieting — or let's call it the "D" bomb — is a lose-lose situation. You lose self-esteem as your body suffers from the rise and fall of pounds. In the end you're ashamed of yourself because you're right back where you started. You just can't beat the science of your body, so let's work WITH it.

We are dealing with your history — emotionally, biologically, psychologically, all of it. As a result of your history, you have a hormone scenario, very personally yours. This super foods program heals your body and balances your hormones (which are responsible for your cravings).

Let's focus on what you can and should have — really good whole, organic food in energy-building combinations. Super foods heal the body by reducing inflammation. Inflammation is the precursor to all illness and aging. Watch your skin begin to glow and enjoy the calm, peaceful feeling within; enjoy the extra energy and the desire to smile. You will see and feel a difference as you rebuild your body with super foods. It is possible to look and feel better than you ever have. Here's the game. Just GET IT IN.

> Ask yourself: Is it Fresh? Organic? Life-giving? Colorful? Made by God or Mother Nature?

If the answer to those is yes, it's a go. You need it. Get it in your body. Enjoy it. Chill it, season it, blend it and make it tasty. It's important to really enjoy good food.

> *Physical fitness is not only one of the most important keys to a healthy body, it is the basis of dynamic and creative intellectual activity.*
> — John F. Kennedy

Week 3

This Week's Assignments:

- Practice facial posturing exercise daily.
- Focus on walking posture. Practice at all times.
- Exercise at least 4 times this week, 55–70 minutes each session, followed by 15–20 minutes of stretching and meditation.
- Begin food combining.
- Read the "A" List often. Eat and drink as many options from the list as you can each day.

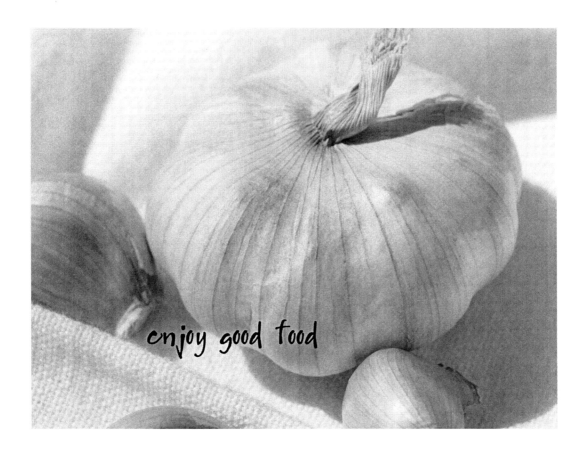

enjoy good food

Continue To:

- Practice meditation 15–30 minutes daily.
- Eliminate toxins from the body. Be aware of all toxic elements, whether thoughts, food, or people around you, and commit to becoming free of them.
- Review your journal writing from Weeks 1 and 2.

Today's date _____

> Every man is the builder of a temple called his body.
>
> — Henry David Thoreau

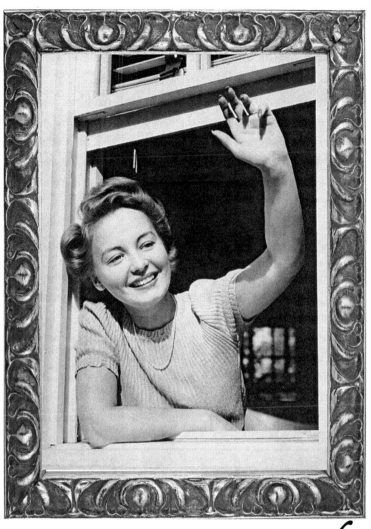

Week 4

This Week's Focus:
Stay Out of Your Own Way
Choices and Setbacks
The Beautiful Body you're Building

They Got the Name Right

Getting back to my friend Janet's serendipitous meeting with Steve McQueen — as the kids in the classroom spread the misconstrued information around like down feathers in a wind storm ... at least they managed to get his name right. Information on fitness, nutrition, beauty, and wellness trickles down and spreads like rumors, but some of what you know and practice may be right.

It's time we get to the real truth about beauty and health. You have the answers inside and instinctively know more than you think about the style of living that works for you. The personal truths you have not yet discovered will be revealed within your journaling. Once you have gone through this program step by step, it will be a powerful tool for you for many years to reread and discover more about the evolution of your genuine self.

Stay Out of Your Own Way

Feeling great has its own gravitational pull. I hope you feel wonderful about the positive changes in your body, disposition, and relationships — this is a reward for your bravery and commitment. If you feel thinner, calmer, happier, more in charge of your life, or notice other improvements — great! That's exactly what we're aiming for because this awareness will cause you to want more. Your body has intelligence, and it wants to feel good and to heal itself — THAT is its natural function and what it does best[1]. Keep your mind open to possibilities, and watch for more positive changes in your body and health. Your body will continue to reveal its amazing capabilities.

We are reconstructing your lifestyle, and this calls for replacing old beliefs and addictive patterns of behavior with habits that create fulfillment, personal power, and a strong, beautiful body. Relationships, people around you, and life's events can bring about emotions of all sorts, but the only person capable of derailing your path of improvement is YOU. Sometimes you need to simply GET OUT OF YOUR OWN WAY. Albert Einstein said it beautifully; "A human being is a part of a whole, called by us 'universe,' a part limited in time and space. He experiences himself, his thoughts and feelings as something separated from the rest ... a kind of optical delusion of his consciousness. This delusion is a kind of prison for us, restricting us to our personal desires and to affection for a few persons nearest to us. Our task must be to free ourselves from this prison by widening our circle of compassion to embrace all living creatures and the whole of nature in its beauty."

If our thoughts have held us hostage, then it is our task to free ourselves from our own prison.

Old, harmful behaviors are driven by your old way of thinking and way of life. Even detrimental habits can feel comfortable simply because they are familiar, so

---

1. Sanders, Jerry. "Healing Intelligence." Jerry Sanders Kinesthetic Healer. 5 July 2009. www.readingthebody.com/healing-intelligence.

watch for them. They may rear their ugly heads from time to time. Make sure you aren't the one getting in your own way.

You "Get in Your Own Way" at Times like These:

If any of these apply to you, highlight or place a sticky tab in this page and refer to the "instead" suggestions often.

Eating when bored or emotionally upset

INSTEAD:
- *Stay with the emotion you are feeling for a few moments.* Try to discover why it is there. Boredom may actually be loneliness. The upset feeling (stress) may be nervousness or anger, causing you to feel out of control. In the past you used food for comfort, as something you could control. Recognize the old emotion. Take a minute to understand how this landed in your psyche.
- *Acknowledge that habitual eating will only exacerbate your problems by causing excess weight, low self-esteem, toxic feelings, and ultimately, disease.* Storing this negative emotion in your body connects it to your thoughts and starts the muddy kickball "bouncing around inside your house" again, preventing you from healing. Your body will have to work overtime to digest the unnecessary food, store it in fat cells, and then carry that extra weight with you everywhere you go. And there goes the vicious cycle. If you can identify this emotion — the one driving you to rifle through the kitchen cupboards — then and only then will you have a shot at truly releasing it.

Physical compulsive behaviors — grinding teeth, twitching, nail-biting, hair-twirling, foot-tapping, fast talking or rambling words, etc.

INSTEAD:
- *Take a deep breath and bring your awareness back into your body.* Feel the energy of your body. Discover the underlying need that causes you to keep expending energy needlessly. It may be discomfort or nervousness from past worries. Pinpoint where it comes from. Stress focused into physical behaviors (the teeth, the foot, etc.) diminishes your ability to feel peace and balance. These movements can cause unnecessary damage and block the total energy flow of your body. This

restricts your mind from being open and calm because it is busy wrangling this movement.

- *Find the trouble area and soften it, then stop. Breathe into it as you hold the word "peace" in the front of your mind. Take a slow deep breath and allow the behavior to subside.*

Having a dislike for exercise

INSTEAD:

- *Feel appreciation for your body and the gift of movement.* Your former belief system may have thought of exercise as hard work or a bother. Now you will find joy in movement by focusing on your body. Your body craves your attention. It is the one machine that improves with use. By working the mind and body in synergy with movement, you'll increase oxygen to all parts of your body, gain muscle tone, have a clearer thought process, release toxins, gain a leaner and more disease-resistant body, and have the energy to move around and enjoy life to its fullest. That's when your body will begin to crave exercise because, in actuality, it really loves it.
- *Bring to mind the gift your body is and all the miracles it performs daily to keep you going.* Bring to mind a function you have not appreciated before such as hands that can grip, the creation of tears to protect your eyes, blood that is continually purified, muscles being repaired around the clock, an injury from the past that has healed — the list is endless. Try to think of something new and feel love deep inside for your amazing body. Take a slow deep breath as you meditate on this function or body part for a moment.

Stumbling Blocks

Circle the the stumbling blocks that seem to be in your path. Then, on the line beneath each one, make plans to step over or around that block:

1. Eating late at night.
   - My plan:

_____

_____

_____

_____

_____

2. Returning to sugar and sweet foods.
   - My plan:

_____
_____
_____
_____

3. Not having enough meal time preparation.
   - My plan:

_____
_____
_____
_____

4. Not feeling motivated.
   - My plan:

_____
_____
_____

5. Feeling overwhelmed and having trouble staying focused.
   - My plan:

_____
_____
_____
_____

6. Eating too much food at meal times.
   - My plan:

_____
_____
_____
_____

7. List here any other old, physical habits that may cause you to get in your own way.

_____
_____
_____
_____
_____
_____
_____

What's Luck got to Do with It?

Your body tells a complete story about the way you live and how you take care of yourself. Your facial expression, your posture, your weight, the way you move — all reveal information about you. Every food you eat dictates how your body feels. If you want to look special, you must take special care of yourself.

Over the years I have been continually asked, "How does Racquel Welch (or Sandra Bullock, Jennifer Aniston, or whoever is the celebrity of their choice) get her skin to look like that? What does she do to look so radiant and beautiful?" The answer frustrates many who hope for a quick fix, a product they can buy or a miracle treatment. The answer is, "Her maintenance program and grooming ritual." She carefully chooses her cosmetics, her foods, her drinks, and the exercise she gets. Everything is strategically planned. The result is her star-powered appearance.

Sure, there are a few jet-setters in their twenties, burning the candle at both ends and still managing to look good with a couple of hours of grooming. Check back with them in a few years; I guarantee it'll catch them. Mark my words, there's no free lunch. There are good genes, but with the right care even those who did not get the best from the gene pool can look like a celebrity and feel like an athlete.

Feeling "lucky" is as far away from stress and anxiety as you can get. These emotions are polar opposites. Allowing positive thoughts to flow through you keeps the physical body at peace and your bodily functions running smoothly. When the body feels a sense of peace, it can achieve balance. Your entire being is an intricate arrangement of systems working together to achieve equilibrium. Therefore, balance is synonymous with good health.

We now know that negative emotions[2] bring aging and illness to the body[3]. If you are a critical person and optimism and positive thoughts don't come naturally, you may be pleasantly surprised by the unexpected changes coming your way. Because you have released toxic emotions that were stored in your body, your perspective will naturally shift. You will see things from a different point of view. You may have less of a propensity to gossip and criticize others. Your mind will be more open to new processes and ideas because you have a clear environment for positive thoughts and creative ideas to develop.

If negativity was a learned behavior for you, it's time to let it go so the "Authentic You" can emerge. It may be difficult to avoid family members or friends who easily find fault in others, but if you can't steer clear of them, you can artfully change the subject. When you release critical, judgmental thoughts, you allow your mind to have creative ideas. Now is the time to pick up a writing tablet or paintbrush or start a sewing project, and see what happens!

"Feeling Lucky" Meditation

- Begin practice of this exercise daily. This takes about one minute, and there is bang for your buck in the return:
- In the morning (any time of day is fine, but morning is best), preferably in a quiet place, stand up straight with your spine aligned, chest open and shoulders relaxed. Close your eyes. Take a deep, full breath then exhale slowly and completely. With the next breath, focus on what in your life makes you feel lucky or grateful. What is there in your life that you feel wonderful about? What do you consider to be a great blessing or the greatest gift you have?
- Whatever it is, bring it to mind and stay with it. Identify it in your mind for a few breaths; breathe it into your body. Rather than just think about it, let the lucky or grateful feeling come over you; **breathe it into your body.** Draw that feeling in with the breath. Let the breathwork be relaxed and full for a while. For the last few breaths of this exercise, take your awareness into your body. Feel appreciation for your body; feel gratitude for the health you have, no matter what its current state may be. Have appreciation for a body that can take you from place to place and allow you to do all that you do; it has brought you to this place. Breathe that in. Stay here for a few breaths. Open your eyes when you are ready.

---

2. Chopra, Deepak. Ageless Body Timeless Mind. New York: Harmony Books, 1993.
3. Mercola, Joseph. "Negative Emotions Can be Deadly to your Health." 13 January 2007. www.articles.mercola.com/sites/articles/archive/2007/01/13/negative-emotions-can-be-deadly-to-your-health.aspx.

Oh Baby

The first thing you learned to do after you were born was to eat. More than just hunger, a primal urge drives us to eat. For the first few years of our lives it was pretty much all that mattered. We awakened our parents at night by crying for a bottle. Later on we had to have "patty cake, patty cake" before taking a bite of peas. And heaven forbid, that a child would play a game of soccer without a sweet treat afterward … and the list goes on. Food is everywhere, connected to most events in our lives. Since we schedule our lives around three square meals a day, many of our habits are traditionally woven around food.

Same Stuff — Different Day.

The average American eats between eight and ten different meals; they are just interchanged. We like what we like because we are comforted by it, used to the taste sensation, have easy access to it, or have connected a form of pleasure to how it makes us feel. List here 5 meals you have over and over:

_____

_____

_____

_____

I have several friends who are rocket scientists at the Jet Propulsion Laboratory (JPL) in La Canada, California. I have enjoyed learning from their experiences of landing the lunar rovers. If there is a problem that may involve saving lives or millions of dollars way out in space with their rover or space ship, they go to every source they have. They look to every possible root for help. The main thing they rely on is CREATIVITY. So it goes for your own body. If there is a problem, a system out of balance, an injury or emotional upset, your body also relies on creativity. It uses all of its own intelligence and capabilities, drawing from all resources of nutrition and healing to bring balance back to your body.

Eating the same foods over and over limits the healing powers of your body. If you have only accumulated nutrients from your favorite foods in a few different meals, your body is at a big disadvantage. It has nowhere to go to find what it needs for healing and rebuilding, even though it may be capable. Your body is continually in the process of rebuilding and renewing itself, and when it has what it needs, aging or breaking down is slowed and sometimes brought to a standstill.

When it is starving for nutrients, as most American bodies are, it shows by aging rapidly.

List three fruits or vegetables you would like to eat more of that you rarely purchase.

_____

_____

List here three fruits or vegetables you've never had that you would like to try.

_____

_____

A Win—Win Situation

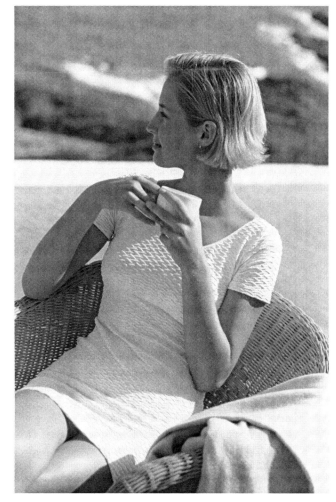

Rather than being driven by habit, make conscious choices that promote optimum health and star-powered beauty. Feeling pressured to "break" a habit puts you in a deprived state, and no one is happy there. Let's focus instead on replacing old bad habits with new choices that will bring rewards. When you look, feel, think, and sleep better, you are excited to continue. These rewards motivate you to make more good choices. As you do, your new habits begin to feel comfortable and natural to you. This brings the bonus of wanting what you need!

No guilt or feeling of restriction is present when

you are wanting what is good for you. It's a win-win situation, and that is when you begin to really live in your lean, strong body.

The Persona Of Thin[4]
From my column "All Health's Breaking Loose"

Years ago as a young mother of small children, I was looking for the "perfect diet" to help me lose a few pounds. When my mother heard about this she said, "Loa, if you want to be thin, you've got to THINK THIN. It's as simple as that." I thought, "Yeah right, Mom."

I didn't think much of it at the time. But now some 30 years later, I realize she knew a very big secret. The masses have searched for this secret only to be eluded, for it is truly a "forest for the trees" scenario. Hundreds of weight-loss products and facilities abound, but the most essential ingredient might already be available to you. Natural slenderness is accompanied by a state of mind. Adopt this state of mind and your body will follow suit.

Let me explain it this way: thin people have a different attitude towards food than those who are overweight. When carrying extra pounds, you see it every time you look in the mirror. Every bite of food you take is considered for its calories and whether or not it is good or bad for you. "Did I eat too much? … Maybe I should have left out the butter … How long until the next meal? … What shall I snack on this afternoon?" It becomes an obsession and truly takes over our thoughts. Since we are surrounded by food in our daily lives, this obsession never really goes "out of mind." It becomes a monster.

Here's where the guilt comes in. The guilt can weigh you down more than the extra pounds. This vicious pattern begins in your head. But, when you are able to get "out of your head" and truly recognize how your body feels and functions, you give yourself a "thinner" way of thinking. Thinner thinking creates a thinner body, and the best part is that this thinner body is free from the torment of the food preoccupation.

---

4. McMorris, Megan. Eight Secrets of the Naturally Slim." Prevention. September 2007. www.prevention.com/cda/article/8-secrets-of-the-naturally-slim/2a2468f271903110VCM10000013281eac_/weight.loss/strategies.for.success.

I have been collecting my own personal research on this concept for years. I was thrilled to learn that official studies are bringing forth some enlightening data as well. Dr. David L. Katz, MD, an associate professor at Yale University, has conducted research on the lives of naturally slender people. Dr. Katz says, "Thin people have a relaxed relationship with food. Those who are overweight, however, tend to be preoccupied by it … mealtime is always on the brain."

The good news is that "thin" behavior can be learned. You can practice being thin by adopting the habits of a naturally slim person. As you do, you restructure your thinking. Here are the secret habits to a thin persona. I'll refer to The Naturally Slender as TNS.

TNS recognize that hunger is not urgent. Many of us think of hunger as a terrible thing to be avoided and we may eat more often just so we never have to feel that hunger. When our stomach is empty we think, "I need something to eat and I need it right now!" Thin people don't mind feeling a little hungry; they know there is another meal coming at some point and don't pay much attention to a growling stomach. They view hunger pangs as a normal function — your body's way of looking out for you — and a gentle reminder, not a cry for help.

TNS dislike the feeling of "full." They don't worry about cleaning their plates and would rather be satisfied than stuffed. When you've eaten lightly, enjoy feeling energetic and mobile after mealtime. Focus on how easy it is to get around and how great it is to feel perky because you have fueled your body with just enough.

TNS eat more fresh food. A 2006 study published in the Journal of the American Dietetic Association reports that lean people eat more fruit. On average, thin people have one more serving of fruit per day than overweight people do. They also have less fat and more fiber in their diets. High-calorie processed foods add strain to the body and bog down the digestive system. Fresh fruits, vegetables, and whole grains nourish the body, reduce cholesterol and bring you energy. Studies show that overweight people eat less fresh food than their thinner counterparts.

TNS get enough shuteye. A study from Eastern Virginia Medical School says that thin people sleep two more hours per week (about 17 minutes per day) than those who are overweight.

One of the hormones released during sleep is leptin. Leptin is produced by fat cells that signal the degree of hunger to the brain. Lack of sleep is associated with lower levels of this appetite-suppressing hormone. Sticking to a regular bedtime helps to ensure you'll get enough Z's.

TNS have other outlets for their emotions. Rather than turning to comfort foods when feeling emotional, they have more options. Calling or e-mailing a friend helps when lonely, walking to the park or through the mall can squelch boredom, exercise, such as jogging, is great for frustration or tension, and stretching, such as yoga, relieves stress. Thin people turn to food less often than those who are overweight.

TNS don't have a quantity issue. Thin people don't buy into "the more the merrier" concept when it comes to food. They don't worry about getting "super sized"; they are content with their routine and tend to be predictable when it comes to food choices. They often choose to eat from smaller dishes.

TNS move more. The Mayo Clinic reports that thin people are on their feet for an additional two and a half hours per day. In one year's time this translates to 33 pounds that have been burned off. They sit less than the rest of us and are more likely to take the stairs or walk instead of drive. Find reasons to move around your home or office, and be the first one up to get the door or phone. Moving around is productive, makes you feel dynamic, and will help you become thinner. And the thinner you become, the more you'll feel like moving — this is the kind of cycle we want.

No matter what gene pool you have, the bottom line is that your relationship to food predicts the size of the jeans you wear. Attachment to food is a learned behavior and it can be unlearned. By practicing the secrets of thin people, we can reinvent our own way of thinking. When you act like a thin person, you are retraining your mind to override the body's compulsive eating behaviors. The change in your body will delight you. Think thin and you'll be thin. I guess Mom was right after all.

End of Column

Move It Or Lose It

This week we add a wonderful warm-up to your fitness routine, as shown below. Use this sequence as a warm-up to your workout, and practice it as you arise in the morning on the days you don't exercise. It is designed to clear your mind, awaken your body, and get your vital energy flowing.

Release all your busy thoughts. Breathe in and exhale slowly, allowing the abdomen to rise with the inhalation and fall as you exhale. Focus on your body and listen to your breath. Flow from one posture smoothly into the next.

Warm-Up Routine

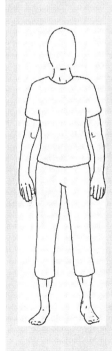

1. Stand with your feet the same width apart as your hip sockets, with toes forward. Lift up out of the pelvis, tuck the chin into the chest slightly, and lengthen up to the ceiling with the crown of your head. With arms down at your sides, roll the palms out and away from the body and drop your shoulders.

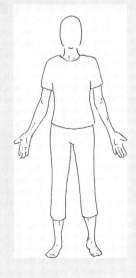

2. With arms straight, lengthen towards the floor and then begin breathing in.

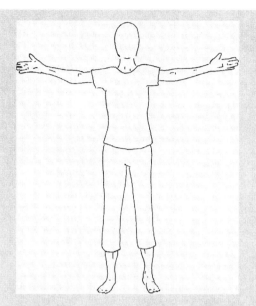

3. Extend arms outward slowly, continuing with a slow breath in, as your arms come all the way up. Reach your hands away from your body.

4. Continue upward until the insides of your arms are by your ears, your arms are straight and your shoulders are low.

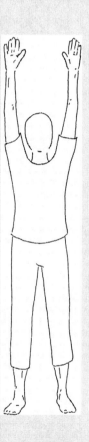

5. Keep your ribs lifted, and exhale as you reverse the move slowly until your hands are back down by your sides.

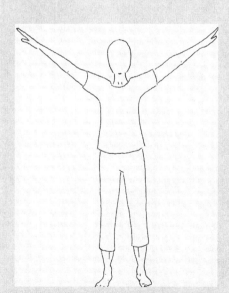

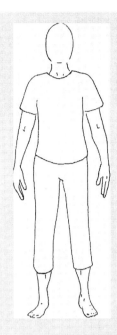

6. Relax for a breath, release your thoughts, and repeat.

7. The third time the arms come up, bring the palms together and interlace the fingers.

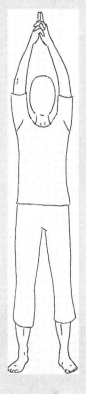

8. Release the index finger and breathe in.

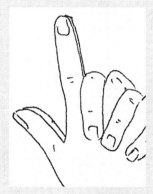

9. Exhale as you push the hips out to one side. Remember to keep your arms straight and your shoulders stacked, so your chest faces forward. Hold here for a few abdominal breaths, come up slowly with a deep breath in, and exhale down on the other side. Repeat.

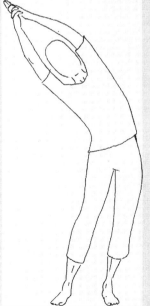

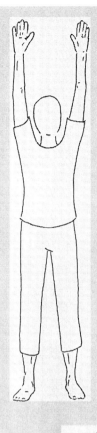

10. After the second set, come back to center with your arms up overhead.

11. Release the hands slowly as if they are floating apart.

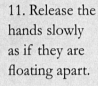

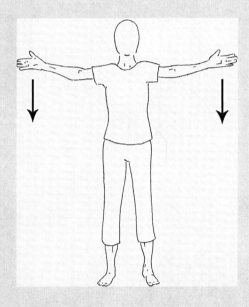

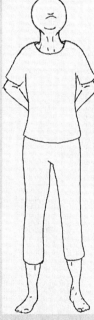

12. Place the hands on the small of your back, palms to the skin. Keep your lower back steady, and gently let your head fall back as you lift your ribs.

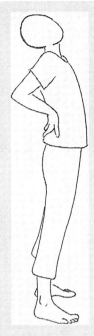

13. Peel the chest open and push the elbows and shoulders back. Hold here for a few breaths, and then focus on your sternum (breastbone) and lift it up towards the ceiling. Press up with your upper chest and be careful not to bend from your lower back. Hold for a few breaths.

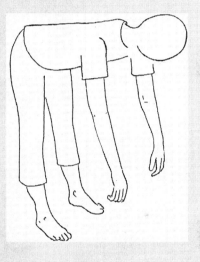

14. Slowly bring your upper body forward from the hips with your back flat and your abs drawn in. Bend all the way down.

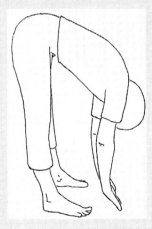

15. Release your arms to the floor and relax your head and neck. Keep your legs straight and abs drawn in as you "hang" there and breathe.

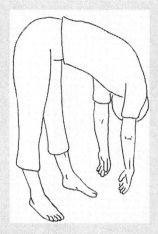

16. Keeping your legs straight, gently swing your arms and body back and forth, warming the low back. After a few breaths, stop in the center and feel the stretch coming up the backs of your legs. Shake your head back and forth as if saying "No," then up and down as if saying "Yes." Release all the neck tension.

17. Bending your knees slightly, take your awareness into your spine, aligning it as you come up slowly, rolling the body up one vertebra at a time until you come back to the beginning posture. Lift up out of the hips, open your chest, roll your shoulders back, and use your shoulder blades to hold there.

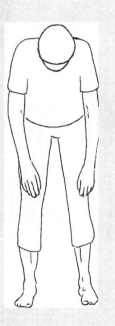

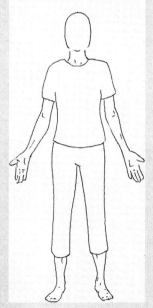

18. Tuck your chin into your body, turn the palms of the hands outward, and tuck your pelvis under slightly. Hold for a few breaths as you clear your mind and bring your awareness into your body. Feel appreciation for your health. Release.

Setbacks

You have been brave in making some necessary changes in your life up to this point, and you should feel good about yourself for doing so. We all have times when we find ourselves in situations that bring about a setback. Part of this process is understanding the areas where you need to be especially careful.

My mother was a baker, and she taught me to love sweets. I was a sugar addict for years before I realized what it was doing to my body. A few weeks after I stopped eating sugar, a good friend of mine (not knowing I had quit) stopped by with my favorite kind of cookie that she had just baked for my birthday. I didn't have the heart to tell her that I couldn't have any of it. She had done such a nice thing, and the cookies were right out of the oven. So I thought, "I'll just have a little while she's here, and then tomorrow I'll start over."

Well, I had the best of intentions, but there were just enough cookies to keep me in sugar heaven for a few days, and after that I lost focus. I began to feel weak and cranky and soon fell comfortably back into my old habits. That one treat shook me off my path for a couple of weeks! Now that I practice meditation and listen to my body, I would be able to handle a situation like that much better.

Hopefully your setbacks won't be as bad as this one was for me, but in our busy lives there are times when things just don't go according to plan. You might find yourself driving a car full of kids home from a game at dinner time with only enough time for fast food — where even your most careful choice isn't good for your body. Or you may work so late into the evening that you are exhausted and drop into bed without having a moment for your daily meditation. Guilt is not part of your thought process now, so do your best. Choose the healthiest item on the fast food menu and eat a small amount or, as you lay there exhausted, do your meditation before falling asleep. Then forget about it and start fresh, with the goal of taking one day at a time, and remembering to plan ahead for pitfalls and stay out of your own way. Begin the next day with meditation and a cup of detox or herb tea and relax, knowing you'll have more control and be more on top of your game. You are the one in charge of your lifestyle. Set your priorities, and these

> *Do not let what you cannot do interfere with what you can do.*
> *— John Wooden, Hall of Fame college basketball coach*

situations will rarely occur. Meditation is a powerful tool that will bring your focus back.

Life is busy, so here are some "Super Food" meal ideas to help you eat well and enjoy your day. Don't let yourself get hungry. Don't skip meals. Try new foods and have fun creating new taste combinations. You'll discover many more tasty meals than listed here, I'm sure!

Note: All foods (including salad dressings and sauces) should be organic and as close to harvest as possible. Water is not listed, but keep drinking it throughout the day (except at meal times).

Breakfast 1
Upon rising, have one glass of water. Eventually follow this with your choice of fresh fruit, such as two small peaches, a handful of berries, three apricots, an apple, fresh pineapple chunks or grapefruit, etc.

Breakfast 2 post-workout
Have detox or white tea, then another serving of fruit. Twenty minutes later, have a handful of almonds, or occasionally a single serving whole grain carb, like a slice of toast. But, if after exercise you feel hungry, replace fruit and toast with one or two eggs scrambled with onion, garlic, and fresh herbs of your choice.

Mid-morning munchie choices
Think of this as a chance for a nutrition boost.
- Red and yellow pepper strips with hummus dip
- A boiled egg
- Celery with almond butter topped with micro greens
- A shot of wheat grass followed by vegetable juice with fresh ginger
- Smoothie made with mango, blueberries, and pomegranate juice
- Sunflower seeds, walnuts, etc.
- Jicama sticks with lime

Lunch ideas
- Salmon and spinach salad with homemade garlic balsamic vinaigrette.
- Vegetable sandwich on whole-grain bread. This is an invitation to get creative and try lots of amazing outside-the-box combinations. Try roasted red peppers, shredded carrots, horseradish, micro greens, fresh dill or basil, roasted beets,

sprouts, cucumber, roasted eggplant, grilled onion, avocado with fresh cracked lemon pepper … the list is endless. Make a beautiful sandwich, then eat half and see how you feel. You can wrap the other half for later.
- Steamed vegetables with green salad, sprinkled with flax seed.
- Tuna salad with Vegenaise or mayo, loaded with cucumber, dill pickle, onion, and celery served in lettuce cups topped with micro greens
- Sauté garlic, onion, and zucchini in a pan with a few leaves of spinach; scramble with two eggs and fresh seasonings.
- Lentil or vegetable soup, sprinkled with flaxseed
- Shrimp cocktail with micro green side salad

Afternoon snack ideas

Have a handful of almonds and detox, white tea, or herb tea. Then refer back to the midmorning munchie list above, or finish the portion you set aside from lunch!

Dinner Ideas

- Grilled chicken breast, green salad with fresh herb vinaigrette, sautéed kale or spinach with garlic, side of roasted red peppers.
- Baked spaghetti squash topped with marinara sauce made with fresh garlic and herbs, colorful side salad of beets, carrots, or any other favorite vegetables.
- Rosemary chicken, roasted baby grape tomatoes and asparagus, with cucumber salad.
- Eggplant parmesan (unbreaded), sautéed zucchini, and a green salad.
- Baked salmon, roasted sweet potatoes, broccoli, lentils.
- Baked white fish, sautéed spinach with garlic, green salad with avocado, finely julliened red or yellow peppers, sprinkled with flax seeds and vinaigrette.
- Roasted winter vegetable stew, spring green salad with pine nuts, beets, and goat cheese.

More Snack Ideas

- Slice jicama in long julienne pieces, then drizzle with lime. Keep in a container in your fridge and have as much as you like.
- Divide a one-pound bag of organic raw almonds into about 10 small Ziploc baggies. They'll hold about 1½ ounces each. Keep them in the fridge so they're handy to take on the run. Have one in your purse, your car, and at your desk.
- Freeze blueberries in small baggies. Have in the afternoon or two hours after eating. They are nature's mini popsicles.
- Albacore tuna with Vegenaise, celery, and fresh cracked lemon pepper stacked on cucumber slices.

- Dip zucchini sticks in hummus.
- Spread almond butter on celery sticks (avoid peanut butter for now).

Evening treats
- Hot bath.
- "A" List tea of your choice, or ginger or chamomile tea.
- Foot self-massage.
- Frozen blueberries or grapes (use this option if you've had an early dinner, 6 pm or earlier. Any fruit or juice must be two hours after dinner).
- Martini glass of green juice, mangosteen juice, or pomegranate juice.
- A handful of pumpkin seeds, sunflower seeds, or walnuts.
- Fresh cherries, cantaloupe, or the best-looking seasonal fruit you can find.
- Anything from the "A" List

As you discover other favorites that meet your new standards, list them here.

_____

_____

_____

Tips for Dining Out
- Decide what you should eat and order it prepared the way you want it — without reading the menu.
- Feel regal — there's no need to clean your plate. Take home half. Put it in a container before you start eating.
- Food combining in a restaurant just takes asking. Smile at the waiter and request a side veggie instead of the nasty white bread he wants to give you. Most places are on board with this now because of the low-carb craze. Ask for what you want. They can hold the croutons or salad dressing — just ask.
- Stay out of franchises — there are far too many additives that you cannot see or control. You have a better chance of getting simply prepared, less toxic food in a locally owned and operated café or restaurant.

Proteins Needed
Nuts * seeds * beans * olives * avocados * lean organic chicken & fish* * soybeans (fresh only. Avoid all soy products unless certified organic.) * red meat (in moderation).

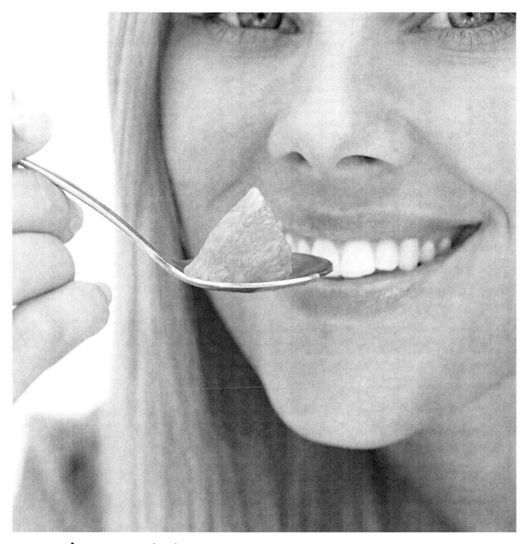

Starches Needed
Potatoes * pumpkin * yams * squash * carrots* parsnips * artichokes * peas * lentils * wild rice * whole grains * whole-wheat pasta * beans * beets (try to incorporate as many super foods, such as beets and yams, as possible)

Use These Fats
Olive oil * butter * cream

Cheese and Nuts
These are part fat and protein. For our purposes count them as a protein.
REMINDER: READ THE LABELS. CHOOSE ONLY ORGANIC FOODS.

Go Easy On

Cheese * red meat * eggs * pure honey * pure maple syrup * dates * figs * raisins * prunes — especially while trying to lose weight

Tips

- If you feel hungry, drink a glass of water to make sure that hunger is really what you are feeling. Be careful not to get dehydrated.
- Eat raw unsalted nuts between meals. They feed the satiety center of the brain and help to release hormones that make you feel satisfied and keep you from getting hungry.
- Relieve your pantry of toxic temptations.
- Set aside time for beautiful meals. Sit on your patio, use your favorite dishes and placemats, and relax.
- Avoid eating when rushed or stressed.

This week's assignments:

- Have the intention to get out of your own way.
- Plan and experiment with vegetarian meals.
- Practice the seven-step warm-up daily as you arise in the morning. Add it to the beginning of your workout as well.
- Exercise a minimum of 4 days this week. Each session should be 60–75 minutes long.

Continue to:

- Delete toxic emotions from your life. Use your journal for this when needed.
- Practice the "feeling lucky" meditation daily.
- Be aware of your self and your habits.
- Meditate 15–30 minutes daily.
- Delete toxic foods from your life.
- Review your journal.
- Practice walking posture at all times.
- Combine your foods, reviewing guidelines when necessary.

Today's date _____

Take care of your body.
It's the only place you have to live.

— Jim Rohn

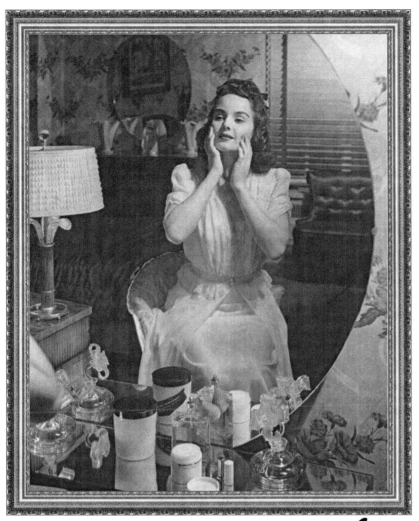

Week 5

This Week's Focus:

Feeling Beautiful
Your New Body Image
Be your own Makeup Artist
Eyebrow Shaping and Skin Care

Every woman is beautiful and every man is handsome — even if they don't know it yet. If they don't know it, it's because they aren't aware of their true potential. To be beautiful, handsome, or even strikingly gorgeous, first you must feel it. Once you feel it, it's only a matter of a few simple skills.

Eight-year-old Sally came home from school with a frown. She said, "Momma, I'm not pretty like the other girls. They all have bows in their hair." Sally's mother was poor, so she cut a piece of white ribbon from a dress of her own. The next day before school, she tied up Sally's ponytail with the ribbon. Sally felt so pretty, she skipped off to school. A few days later, Sally's mother could not find the ribbon. Not having any other ribbon, she only pretended to tie a bow in her daughter's ponytail. She didn't have the heart to tell Sally it was gone. When she got home from school Sally said, "It's a good thing I have this bow in my hair, because now I'm pretty like the other girls!"

Little Sally believed the ribbon made her pretty. Even when the ribbon was lost, she still felt pretty because she believed it was there.

The Titanic Learned it the Hard Way

Our minds are like icebergs. The part that thinks it's in control, or the conscious part, is what peaks above the surface. But it amounts to only about 25 percent of the total iceberg. Just as they learned on the Titanic, there's much more to this than meets the eye. The other 75 percent, or the much larger "subconscious" mind, lies tucked quietly under the surface[1]. No one else has your personal history. It is kept with you in thoughts and memories, accessed through your mind. With each of these thousands of thoughts and memories came emotion and those feelings are stored throughout "you." They become part of your biology. All the systems of your body work together to form one whole person, so those emotions are stored not only in your conscious mind but throughout your body in organs, muscles, connective and soft tissues. Like the submerged portion of the iceberg, this information is not generally recognized by the part of the iceberg on the surface, or our conscious intellect. But it's there, causing us to feel and react according to past experiences.

Every cell in your body has intelligence, and even when the conscious mind is not aware of it, their memory banks are storing the data that creates your disposition, personality, ability to love, self-esteem, and so much more[2]. Have you ever heard someone describe a time when they were really sick to their stomach and they said, "Just thinking about it makes me feel sick"? With only their thoughts, they are capable of re-creating that former physical state. Likewise, recalling the feeling of falling in love brings a sense of bliss and slows the heart rate. As we think, so we are. The emotions we store and carry around day after day, and year after year, create the physical body we walk around in.

1. Chopra, Deepak. Ageless Body Timeless Mind. New York: Harmony Books, 1993
2. Albrecth-Buehler, Guenter. "Cell Intelligence." 9 July 2009. www.basic.northwestern.edu/g-buehler/summary.htm

Body Memory Meditation

Close your eyes, clear your mind and relax your breath. Let your awareness take you to a time when you were at your most strong and energetic self. Remember what you could do physically. Visualize your young body and remember how it felt to be active and strong with boundless energy. Allow the details of the dance troupe you were in, the baseball games you played, a touchdown you ran, or the drill team you marched with to come to mind. Remember the moves and music. As you breathe, bring this vitality into your body. Stay here until your breath has slowed. Draw in a breath of gratitude and feel thankful for your body and all the gifts it brings to your life. Exhale slowly and smile before opening your eyes.

- Each day take a few moments to recall your lean strong body, how it looked and felt, and the surroundings — the grass or gymnasium, tennis court or field. Visualization helps access body memory, and with practice, becomes a powerful tool that keeps us in touch with the performance of our bodies. Visualization allows our mind and body to work in synergy.

At any given moment, our state of health reflects the sum total of our beliefs since birth. Our society wholeheartedly embraces many ridiculous notions and touts them as gospel — ideas like "turning 50 means you're old," "being wealthy means you're smart," "being a celebrity makes you admirable." We can choose to not get "sucked in" to this ridiculousness and find authenticity instead.

As a personal trainer, I often hear, "Well, now that I'm 30 (or 40 or 50), I guess it's normal to have aches and pains." These words are nails on a chalkboard to me. By expecting degeneration, you set up a self-fulfilling prophecy. This idea brings feelings that will prepare your body for breakdown and the reality of the aches and pains.

All living things respond physically to what they perceive is their reality. If you tie a baby elephant to a stake by his ankle, he will circle around the stake and just keep walking in circles. When he is grown and the bondage has been removed, he will continue to walk in circles. Even though he could take off in any direction he pleased, he doesn't know he is free to roam. The elephant has been conditioned through his experiences, just as many of us have been. Like him, we could take off in a new direction if we pleased. We can certainly be sure the events of our childhood set the stage for our beliefs about ourselves and our experience, and therefore our health. In order to change or improve our reality and state of health, first we must change our beliefs about what is possible. Once we release destructive, unconscious patterns, the body can change. You can have the body you have always wanted to have. It is possible to look and feel better than you ever have before. Rather than expect it to decline, let your body reveal what it is capable of. You might be pleasantly surprised.

Your White Ribbon

In Week One we discussed internal programming and the verbal conditioning that came part and parcel with your upbringing. Your thoughts create your words, your words create beliefs, and just as Sally's experience demonstrated, beliefs structure the beauty you convey. No matter how discouraged you have felt about your face, body or sense of style in the past, it is time to reclaim all the natural beauty you possess and bring it to light.

Negative verbal conditioning limits your capabilities but, over the last four weeks, your search for the "authentic you" has revealed untapped potential within you. Real beauty comes from truly enjoying who you are, feeling great, being optimistic about the possibilities in your life, and then having star-powered grooming skills to help the "Authentic You" shine. You can be as beautiful as you want to be. Your potential is limitless. It's time we found what makes you feel like "the white ribbon is in your hair."

When in your life did you feel the most vital and desirable?
_____

What made you feel this way?
_____
_____
_____
_____

More details — how old were you, and where did you live? How much did you weigh?
_____
_____
_____
_____
_____

How was your life different then from now?

_____

_____

> We can't solve problems by
> using the same kind of thinking
> we used when we created them.
> — Albert Einstein

Body Image

My first job as a makeup artist was on *The Donny & Marie Show*. The show had been a huge success the previous season, and things in preproduction became hectic. Even though I had few secretarial skills, I found myself helping out in the office. In front of my desk was a long, open hallway, so I had a front row seat to watch everyone walk up and down this corridor. This "catwalk" became a visual lesson in body types and postures. I became friends with Kerri, the producer's executive secretary. She was a tall brunette, about sixty pounds overweight. Walking was difficult for her. Carrying the excess weight made her heavy-footed, and, rather than walk, she seemed to trudge slowly down the hall. Kerri suffered from a poor self image. She had been heavy all of her life and seemed to feel as though she was supposed to be heavy, as if everyone expected it from her. She was a people pleaser, and her personal needs were dealt with last.

Kerri fell for a guy and decided it was time to get herself in shape. She was motivated to get his attention and after a few months of crash dieting she had lost more than fifty pounds.

From my front row seat observing her new thin body walk down the hall, it occurred to me that nothing about her movements had changed. She trudged along with a thud in every step, just as she did when she was heavy. Even though she was a much leaner person, her posture and movements had not changed at all.

She seemed to enjoy her "thin time," but it wasn't long before Kerri had gained back all the weight. The way she carried her body demonstrated her internal programming — a signal that she viewed herself as heavy, and even though she could discipline herself to a thinner size, she would have great difficulty breaking out of a lifelong pattern. Disciplining the body into submission with constant restriction while ignoring what goes on inside of us can at best can bring only a temporary modification. Appreciating the lessons in your past experiences, letting go of toxic beliefs and learning to speak the language of your body will guide you to the authentic image of YOU. When this lean, beautiful self image becomes real to you, your new healthy habits feel natural and effortless.

Keep it Real From my column "All Health's Breaking Loose"

Karen wouldn't dream of being a day late for her yearly mammogram. Losing her mother to breast cancer has left her totally committed to her yearly trek to her OB. She feels she should do all she can to prevent herself from contracting the big "C". She also watches her weight in the hopes of staying out of the high-risk category. After her mammogram she meets her girlfriends for lunch. They discuss how dreadful it would be to hear the news of being diagnosed with cancer. Over a Cobb salad and diet soda (there's the weight watching), they furrow their brows and sadly imagine how they would get through this terrible ordeal if it came their way.

I'm not a big fan of chit-chatting about the "what ifs" of the big "C" so let's chat about the big "R," reality. Here's the reality of Karen's day so far: An annual dose of radiation does not reduce your chances of getting cancer. The cost of cancer treatment in the U.S. has almost hit $100 billion per year[3] and this tells us the disease is far too common to allow ourselves to live in a fantasy world about it. Prevention should be a key strategy and that would include omitting known carcinogens such as nitrates (in the bacon in Karen's salad), MSG (in the salad dressing), and benzene (in her diet soda). As for the discussion that day, experiencing fear through commiseration about a weakness in your body is laying the groundwork for creating a disposition similar to that of living with the illness. Maintaining a calm and peaceful disposition is the cornerstone of feeling beautiful. It also strengthens your immune system and wards off illness — which creates a younger looking body. It all comes down to choices: the choices we make

---

3. Henderson, Lisa. "Practice-Centric Programs to Help Payers and Providers Contain Costs and Improve Patient Outcomes Together." U.S. Oncology. 3 September 2008. www.opspharmacist.com/documents/public/newsupdates/innoventoncology.pdf

when we order lunch, and the thoughts we choose to think about and discuss with our friends.

Yes, a mammogram should be relied on for its real purpose and then discussed with a doctor who cares and is well informed. Early detection creates better odds for treatment and, of course, we all want to do the right thing. Let's keep it "real" and keep sight of the power we have to make our own choices. We can choose to feel authentically beautiful and gain the skills to make it a reality.

End of Column

You Call the Shots

Before I begin grooming a female celebrity for a high-profile interview, I select a specific color palette, organize and set up all the cosmetics I have chosen for her, prep her skin, and remind her to take a few deep relaxation breaths. She may be in the makeup chair for up to two hours. Meanwhile, other professionals have selected her wardrobe, led her in a personalized exercise class, freshly colored and styled her hair — all while a lighting crew is busy preparing to illuminate her uniquely shaped face. Star-powered looks are orchestrated by a team of professionals.

You will have to become the stand-in for your team of professionals as we create your very own star-powered look. I often say to my students, "Be your own best stylist. You can do for yourself precisely what needs to be done. Think as if you were your own personal trainer. Think like your own makeup artist. Think like your own hair stylist!"

> *Consider your time each morning "in camp" as your personal treat. It is your chance to clear your mind of any stagnant thoughts that bog you down and inhibit your progress.*

I see many people, especially women, run into the same big problem over and over. They assume that because they are grooming, whether it's coloring their hair, shaping their eyebrows, applying makeup, styling their hair (or whatever) that they have done a "good" thing. The fact that they have spent money and time means improvement should surely be the result. This misconception is way too common. Makeup, hair coloring, and styling are powerful tools that have impact. And, if used improperly, will have the wrong impact. You can make yourself look tired, old, puffy, and extreme just as easily as you can look your very best. For example, if you are a cool-tone person with blue eyes and a pink undertone to the skin, and you are coloring your hair to a warm golden shade, your skin will appear ruddy and tired. The gold tones will appear brassy and highlight the blemishes in your skin and the circles under your eyes. Without intending to, you can actually make yourself look older!

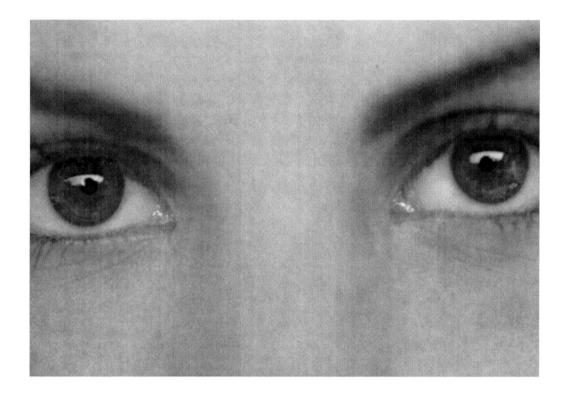

Another personal defrocking of your own beauty comes from overgrooming. Feelings of insecurity or anxiety can bring the compulsion to over-tweeze eyebrows, over-tease hair, apply too much foundation or powder, or use lip liner that's too dark. Rather than focus on the overall picture, we fixate on one thing that we can control. If we stay with it (keep tweezing or teasing or adding more makeup) we can REALLY make it striking, even if it's unflattering.

There is a specific order to this program. Once you have come through Weeks One, Two, and Three, you begin to feel calm and content and many negative habits and compulsions just fall by the wayside. Allow yourself to be free of old habits and accept a fresher style. Let your skin breathe and your hair bounce. This is just one of the many, many perks of allowing your own authentic beauty to emerge naturally.

As your own personal stylist, you can develop the grooming skills necessary to make you look like a star. Your frame of mind is different now, you're more self-aware, and these new realizations help you see yourself more realistically, without bias or old habits popping up. As you study your face and hair and see yourself in a new light, you will find the answers to many questions about your own beauty quotient.

Beauty is a combination of qualities that bring pleasure to the mind or to the senses. Your unique personality, your talents, and your sense of humor are all a significant part of what makes you beautiful. This program is first and foremost about HOW YOU FEEL. Life is a balance of many emotions. If there are insecurities hovering in your heart, now is the time to let them go. When you feel good, toxic emotions such as bitterness, fear, or lack of self-confidence dissipate. When your body feels good, you release insecure thoughts or emotions without even trying. Feeling good overrides insecurity. It's time to feel beautiful so you will BE more beautiful than ever before.

When was the last time you were proud of your appearance?
_____

What created this satisfied feeling?
_____

List at least 10 things you love about yourself that don't have anything to do with the way you look:
_____
_____
_____
_____
_____
_____
_____
_____
_____
_____

You don't have to love all of your physical attributes to feel beautiful. List at least five physical traits about yourself that you love or like.

_____ _____ _____

_____ _____ _____

What activities are you engaged in when you feel strong, competent, and content? List three.

_____ _____ _____

> *No one can make you feel inferior without your consent.*
> *— Eleanor Roosevelt*

Move It. You're in the Way.

We often sabotage our own bodies by clinging to old habits that are comfortable. To fulfill your beauty quotient you will once again have to GET OUT OF YOUR OWN WAY. Here are some examples of getting in the way of being beautiful or handsome. Check the ones that apply to you:

Men and Women: Check the ones that apply to you.

- ☐ I don't want to spend money on my appearance.
- ☐ I don't want to spend time on my appearance.
- ☐ Grooming seems useless because "I can't be beautiful or handsome anyway."
- ☐ I don't trust my own taste and ability to make myself look better.
- ☐ I keep this hairstyle, even though it may be out-of-date or unflattering, because it's easy for me to style.
- ☐ I have changed my face with cosmetic procedures more than once.
- ☐ I furrow my brow, rub my eyes or sleep face down.
- ☐ My hair style might be outdated because I am afraid to try something new.

Women: Check the ones that apply to you.

- [ ] My makeup might be out of date because I'm afraid to try something new.
- [ ] I focus on the application of my makeup or hair (big brows, extreme hair, use of bright colors, over-lined lips) rather than what really reflects my best features. I may borderline on extreme.
- [ ] I waste time by using cosmetics that I don't need.
- [ ] I do not know how to choose colors for my face or hair.

Men: Check the ones that apply to you.

- [ ] I grow facial hair because I'm not sure I want to show my face.
- [ ] I don't want to be accused of leaning toward the feminine, so the only grooming I am used to is haircuts; I haven't ventured into the unknown.

Journal how you might be getting in the way of being beautiful or handsome.

_____
_____
_____
_____
_____

First One on the Set — Put your Best Face Forward

"Setting up" is an important part of a professional makeup artist's job. When on a show, I am the first one to arrive on the set in the morning. Everything must be clean and every cosmetic must be in its place and within reach so application is fast and flawless. I make sure my table is neatly arranged, with no unnecessary clutter, so I can work efficiently. Your makeup should be done as efficiently at home as it is when a celebrity is in the makeup chair. Your time should be spent following your bliss rather than wasted searching through a drawer. If you're wasting 15 minutes each day, that amount of time adds up and can be spent enjoying your family or a hobby.

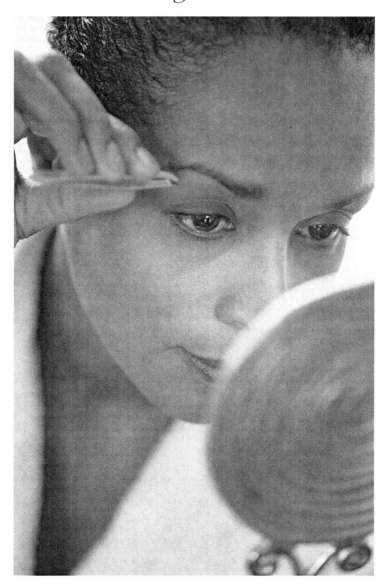

First, choose an area with natural light (an area by a bathroom window is good). Decide what is "your space." Negotiate with family members or roommates if necessary, but make sure that you have a designated drawer, shelf, cabinet or basket that is yours and yours alone. Choose a spot where cosmetics stay clean, and you can add dividers to organize them. Home improvement centers or office supply stores are great places to find drawer organizers. You will need four dividers, one each for face, eyes, lips, and miscellaneous. Be sure to measure your drawer so the dividers fit just right.

Even if you don't use all of these items, organize your cosmetics so the items you use will have a place as follows:

1. Face Compartment:
Foundation, concealer, bronzer, blush, powder, highlighter.

2. Eyes Compartment:
Eye shadows, liner, mascara, tweezers.

3. Lips Compartment:
Lipsticks, lipliners, gloss, lip conditioner.

4. Misc. Compartment:
Small scissors, pencil sharpener, makeup brushes, and applicators.

Keep all cosmetics clean and in their place. Every product has a shelf life and needs to be thrown away when worn-out, broken, outdated, or aged. This does NOT mean when they are all gone. Powdered eye shadows and bronzers become unusable when oil from the sponge tip applicator has picked up moisturizer or body oils from your eye lid or face and touched back onto the shadow. The oil "sets" the powder into the eye shadow container, and the eye shadow will no longer blend smoothly as you apply it. A mascara tube is a moist, warm place — perfect for growing bacteria — and should be replaced every six to eight weeks. Pencils dry out, and all other cosmetics change as they get old, so don't keep them around too long. Keep your makeup fresh.

Do not share your cosmetics, and warn a roommate, sister, or daughter not to raid your drawer.

A magnifying mirror is valuable for checking your application and blending. There are many kinds; usually they are called vanity or magnifying mirrors. Even if your vision is 20/20, mirrors are helpful or even necessary to get a close-up look. A 5X lighted mirror (5 times magnification) mounted at eye level near your makeup drawer will help you achieve professional results.

List here the items you need and specific ways you can improve your grooming area.

I need to get:

_____
_____
_____
_____

I can improve my grooming area by:

_____
_____
_____
_____

What are You Using?

Oh, the power in a bottle of makeup — the promise of youth that comes with a jar of face cream. Whether it's foundation, shampoo, deodorant, body lotion, lip balm, hair gel, mascara, eyeshadow, hair spray, hand cream, body spray or _____ (fill in the blank with the cosmetic item that you use most often), we love cosmetics. We are a high-maintenance grooming culture that lives for the hope of miracles that come from these artfully packaged products. We love the idea of beauty and want to be on the bandwagon, but in order to really be "on that wagon" we need to know what we are actually using.

The FDA regulates this 35 billion-dollar-a-year industry and they certainly have their hands full. During the time it took to write this manuscript, the laws regulating some 10,000 ingredients have changed several times.(footnote #4 goes here) There are many loopholes in state and federal laws that have created a slippery slope for all of us. I encourage you to do some checking on your own behalf. Start with www.safecosmetics.org and see where that takes you. Ask yourself, do you really believe that thousands of chemicals have all been studied individually, collectively, and long-term effects have been determined? It's at this point my mind floats to the state of affairs in Washington, D.C., and the all-too-often sweeping-under-the-rug that affects our daily lives. It is worth a few minutes of your time. Your body's ability to fend off toxins, heal, and become disease-resistant are at stake. Marketing giants would have you only consider — should I choose the red bottle with silver writing, or the blue bottle with gold writing? But you and I know better.

- **Isopropyl Alcohol SD-40** is a very drying, irritating solvent made from a petroleum derivative that strips the skin's natural acid mantle, making us more vulnerable to viruses and bacteria. It ages skin prematurely and promotes brown spots.

- **Phthalates** are used in automotive parts, PVC products, plastic toys and — yes — cosmetics. Rarely identified in ingredient lists, phthalates may be listed as DEP, DBP, and DHEP or even simply as "fragrances." They are endocrine-disruptor chemicals that can damage the heart, lungs, liver, and kidneys, and impair reproduction and development, especially in young males.

- **Mineral Oil** is a petroleum by-product that coats the skin like plastic, clogging the pores. This prevents the skin from doing one of its main jobs: eliminate toxins. It slows down skin function and cell development, which causes premature aging. Manufacturers love it because it's ridiculously cheap. Baby oil is 100% mineral oil with fragrance added. Mineral oil derivatives can be contaminated with cancer-causing Polycyclic Aromatic Hydrocarbons (PAH), such as Paraffin oil, paraffin wax, and Petrolatum.

• **Parabens** such as methyl, propyl, butyl, and ethyl are all preservatives. Known to be highly toxic, they extend shelf life, allowing you to buy a very old product without knowing.

• **Polyethylene Glycol** or PEG compounds are potentially carcinogenic petroleum ingredients that reduce the skin's natural moisture factor. They leave you more vulnerable to bacteria and age the skin. Used in cleansers to dissolve grease and oil, this substance thickens products. It's even in that nasty, gag-inducing spray-on on oven cleaner.

• **Sodium Laureth Sulfate** and **Ammonium Laureth Sulfate**, or SLES and ALES, are good reminders that more than isolating a particular chemical, what matters is the reaction a chemical has when it meets up with other ingredients. Nitrosiamines are a potent class of carcinogens and the result of SLES and ALES combining with other ingredients. Occassionally dressed up with "comes from coconut," these are highly toxic irritants.

• **Sodium Lauryl Sulfate** and **Ammonium Lauryl Sulfate**, or SLS and ALS, are found in most any product that foams. They're even in engine degreasers and garage floor cleaners. Animals that are exposed to SLS or ALS experience eye damage, central nervous system depression, difficulty breathing, severe skin irritation, and even death. SLS and ALS damage the skin's immune system by causing layers to separate and inflame. Can also be disguised as "comes from coconut."

• **Toluene**. For this one I'll only quote a small portion of the Material Safety Data Sheet (MSDS): "Poison! Danger! Harmful or fatal if swallowed. Harmful if absorbed through the skin. Vapor harmful. Flammable liquid and vapor. May affect liver, kidneys, blood system, or central nervous system. Causes irritation to skin, eyes and respiratory tract."… That's only part of the data but I'll stop there[4].

---

4. "Toxic Cosmetics Ingredient List." Alkalize for Health. 14 July 2009. www.alkalizeforhealth.net/ltoxiccosmetics.htm#46

Industry estimates state that an average consumer uses as many as 25 different cosmetic and personal care products containing more than 200 different chemicals each day, but you won't know if any of these are in the products you use unless you turn the bottle over and READ THE LABEL. That's a lot of toxins being inhaled, rubbed in, and absorbed into our bodies. Your body pays the price and the "aroma cocktail" from the layering of fragrances is overwhelming and unattractive. We are a society of "fragrance phobes," and we worry far too much about our personal smells and mask as much of our natural scent as we can. The mixture of perfumes and fragrances leaves us with a heavy and unnatural scent. We each have a body chemistry that is uniquely our own. Rather than work against it by covering it up with heavy perfumes, work with it by finding a natural oil that blends with your own unique smell. Nothing is sexier than being fit and well groomed, with a natural, clean scent — not to mention there may be fewer painful headaches in the future for you and your family.

Choose organic botanical products with essential oils and milder ingredients. It takes a while to find an all-natural product like essential oil in spritz bottles, or mini roll-ons, that work with your personal body scent. Body lotions are easier to replace; you just need to shop in the right stores. Whole Foods and other specialty grocery stores have a great selection. It may take a while to purge through your daily products and get completely switched over to a non-toxic regime, but you can start now with each new purchase you make. It is empowering to know what you are buying and that you can keep these toxic substances out of your home. Allow for trial and error, and don't feel bad if on the first couple of attempts you don't find a product you like. Keep trying until you have an arsenal of safe and effective products you are happy with. Otherwise, you're stuck using ingredients that were poorly studied (or perhaps not studied at all) and sometimes even known to pose serious health risks. Without adequate regulation, these glamorous marketing campaigns will continue to try and get you to buy. It's up to you.

Are You Creating Beauty?

- On a scale of 1 to 10, with 10 being proficient, how confident are you that you can style your own hair and make it look fabulous?
  1   2   3   4   5   6   7   8   9   10
- On a scale of 1 to 10, how confident are you that you can apply your own makeup so that it is flawless and brings out your best features?
  1   2   3   4   5   6   7   8   9   10

- When you shop for cosmetics, how sure are you that you are buying the right thing?

  1   2   3   4   5   6   7   8   9   10

- Are you confident that your current hairstyle is right for you?

  Yes   No   Somewhat

- Are you confident that your current hair color is right for you?

  Yes   No   Somewhat

The Eyes Have It

Gleam + sparkle + twinkle + shine = fabulous. If you have any of these going on, you're probably in good health. Lift your eyebrows or wiggle your ears, and you can feel the delicate muscle structure around your eyes. These thin, delicate orbicularis oculi muscles run in a circle. Unlike your bicep, they cannot be "pumped up." The muscle fibers are softer and need to be treated gently. Pulling or rubbing the eyes can stretch the skin and cause unnecessary wrinkling such as "crow's feet" or under-eye "bags."

This thin skin is only about 20 micrometers thick[5]. Unlike the skin on your hands and feet (which is much thicker), this delicate skin is more sensitive to damage from irritating substances or from being over-stretched.

The eyes are very telling of what's happening inside our bodies. Allergies, anger, aging, and illness all show up first in the eyes, so take note of your eyes on a good day. Notice the bone area above the lid and under your eyes. Any puffiness or swelling will change this line of your face. Puffiness can be a build-up of lymph or too much salt in your diet. If you are prone to under-eye discoloration, it may be caused by slow blood flow or blood vessels showing through the thin skin. Be mindful of changes in your diet and how they affect your "dark circles." Tired, lifeless eyes usually mean your diet needs a "super foods boost." The disposition of your digestive tract shows in your eyes, so make sure you are choosing from the "A" List and eating a variety of fresh organic produce — as fresh from the harvest as possible. Bring the life force from a shot of wheat grass or a fresh-picked piece of fruit into your body, and you'll bring that sparkle back to your eyes. Go ahead and twinkle!

The Most Underrated Feature On The Face

Your eyebrows express what you are feeling and punctuate what you are saying. Imagine trying to show a concerned look of "Can I help you?" or the tender expression of "thank you" to a loved one without them. Many men and women

---

5. Brannon, Heather, M.D. "Skin Anatomy." 9 April 2007. www.dermatology.about.com/cs/skinanatomy/a/anatomy.htm. See also www.cosmeticsdatabase.com.

Tip

Your ring finger is the weakest finger on your hand and should be used when touching the under-eye area. Always work from the outside towards the nose and never pull, rub or stress the under-eye area. The delicate orbicularis oculi muscles run in a circular motion around the eye socket, and working from the outside corner towards the nose supports the muscle and resists sagging. Never pull down or towards the outside of the face. With your ring finger lightly touching the skin, pat and gently move across in a circular motion. Blending eye shadow in this direction also prevents you from following your own arch and "dragging" the eye downward.

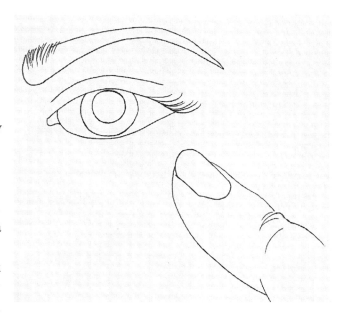

leave them untouched because they just don't know what to do with them. Women commonly report to me, "I've never really done anything with them because I didn't know what to do." So, this is where we start, with the most underrated feature on your face. When shaped properly, your brows give a lift to the eye area and give more presence to the cheek bones. They can make your face look more oval shaped and bring a fresh, perky, and polished finish to your overall appearance. If your eyes are the window to your soul, then the brows must be the drapes!

Here are some guidelines to finding the right shape for you:
- Look straight ahead into a mirror.
- Use a very thin, clean object at least three inches long, like the end of a thin makeup brush or a chop stick.
- Line it up on the outside of your nose, going straight up to the inside corner of your eye.
- This is your inside length. If there are hairs to the inside of the ruler they should be tweezed.

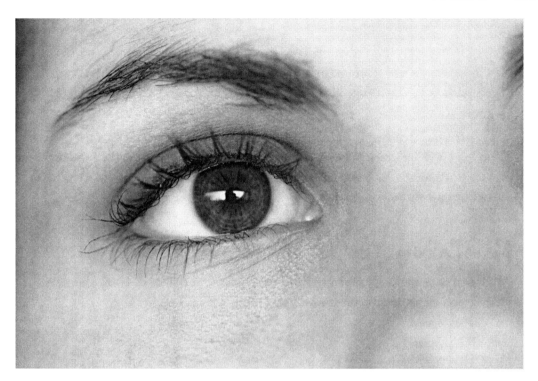

- While still on the side of the nose, lean the chopstick or brush handle to the outside corner of the same eye. Your outside length stops where the ruler intersects the brow. Any hairs beyond the ruler (closer to the hairline or temple area) should be tweezed. If your brow length falls short of this point, lightly fill it in using light feathery strokes of a brow pencil.

To determine your optimum brow shape, carefully consider, "Is my face narrow or wide? Are my eyes close or wide-set? Is my nose narrow or wide?" We want to bring balance to your face. A wide face needs a heavier brow, close-set eyes need slightly more width between brows and a wide nose needs heavier brows with less room between them. Too much tweezed space can create a "fleshy" appearance. Whatever your brow shape is, remember to avoid over-tweezing. It is the most common mistake in eyebrow shaping and can create an unbalanced, fleshy, or harsh look.

Waxing is an alternative I recommend in very few cases. YOU are your makeup artist! There is no need to pay someone for a task you can do so simply yourself. When you defer to the taste of the wax operator, you are no longer in control — she is, and you are at the mercy of her taste. YOU should be the judge. You know your face better than she does, and the time and money saved on paying a technician can be happily spent elsewhere. Shaping brows only takes minutes, and once they are groomed and shaped you only need to maintain them by checking for stray regrowth twice a week or so.

Tip

If tweezing is painful, place an ice cube in a piece of tissue and hold on the area for a few seconds, or apply baby teething gel to the area for a few seconds before starting. This will have a numbing effect, and tweezing will be more comfortable.

If you have a wide or heavy jaw, full lips, or very large eyes, you will need to have a fuller, thicker brow. If your face is delicate and thin, then the brow can be thinner. Once you have determined the appropriate length, it's time to define and shape your brows.

Maintaining the Ultimate Eyebrows

- Keep your tweezers separate from the household tweezers. They should be handy and clean, waiting in your divider bin for EYES.
- Never tweeze eyebrows from the top. The "lift" in the arch refines the bone structure. If you have random facial hairs or light, fine peach fuzz, this can be tweezed from above the arch, but do not tweeze actual eyebrow hairs above the top.
- Tweeze toward the ears, with a quick, outward, plucking action. One hair at a time.
- Tweeze hair in the direction of growth. Never pull a hair from the left brow across towards the right side or from the right brow over towards the left side. This can cause bleeding or make a pockmark.
- To fill in sparse areas and add definition, use a light shade of a sharpened eyebrow pencil in small feathery strokes, working upward toward the arch or

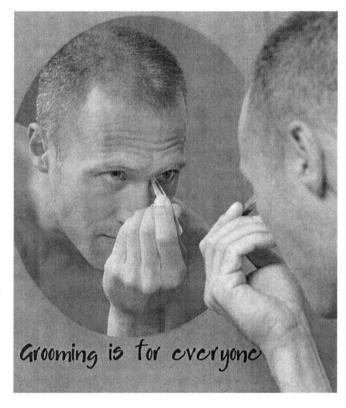

Grooming is for everyone

gently downward to add length. Choose a color slightly lighter than your natural brow color. A blonde pencil can create definition even if you are a brunette. Avoid pencils that are too dark. If in doubt when purchasing, opt for the lighter shade.

- Keep the eyelid free of regrowth and light fuzzy hairs.
- If brows are long or curly, trim using the comb on your eyebrow brush and small, sharp scissors. Comb upward and trim the ends.
- Check the brows for regrowth every other day. Even if there are only one or two hairs, tweeze them so your brows are maintained.

Now that your brows are beautifully shaped, the maintenance is easy. Watch for regrowth. You may have to tweeze one hair one day, none the next, and some days maybe two. It is a simple part of the grooming process that requires your attention but takes very little time. For light or sparse brows, use a pencil in upward, feathery strokes.

Tip
Eyebrow pencils should be kept sharp for definition. In warm weather, the tip can become soft, causing smearing. To get a fresh point, put the pencil in the refrigerator for about 10 minutes before sharpening.

Skin Care
YOUR HABITS AND THOUGHTS HAVE CREATED THE CONDITION YOUR SKIN IS IN RIGHT NOW.

Skin care and makeup application continually evolve, but certain mistakes through the years continue to be troublesome for many people. Over and over the same mistakes are commonly made, so rather than provide you with superfluous pages of information you already know — let's take a simple troubleshooting approach and get right to the most common grooming mistakes. Your comfort zone and personal sense of style are important. But no matter what styles and products you currently prefer, we can make it better by fine-tuning with these hints.

KNOW YOUR SKIN TYPE, and select all your skin care products accordingly. If your skin feels tight after cleansing and needs moisture right away, then your skin is DRY. If you have slight excess shine in the afternoon and prefer a light moisturizer, your skin is in the normal range. If you have a heavy afternoon shine and feel the need to wash your hair daily, then your skin is oily. Notice products that irritate your skin, and use products for sensitive skin when necessary. You may be sensitive around the eyes but not on your face, or maybe you react to added fragrances. Know everything you can about your skin — it's YOUR skin!

CLEANSE LIKE A BIG KID

Use a mild soap appropriate for your skin type and be gentle. Remember forgotten spots that you may not see: right under the chin, along the jaw, on the inside corners of the nose between your eyes, and under your nose. Use a gentle, circular motion going outward toward the hairline. More than just cleaning the skin, the massage brings blood circulation to the face, which boosts collagen production, keeps the skin supple and brings healing to the area.

Think of this as a daily spa treatment that you do for yourself. Be thorough and gentle as you rinse with tepid water. Aging skin should avoid hot water. Pat dry carefully with a soft, white "for face only" cotton cloth or towel. (I recommend white because it is free of dyes and can be washed in hot water.) Keep face cloths separate from other washcloths. Be careful not to rub as this stretches the skin, causing wrinkles. Set down your cloth and take a moment to relax and breathe while you gently pat with the pads of your fingers. Use a quick patting motion, going across the forehead, cheekbones, cheeks and chin area. This skin-toning treatment takes about one minute and should be done daily to keep circulation and collagen production activated.

The basics of beauty are in how you care for your skin, so your skin care ritual needs to be efficient, streamlined, and tailored to your needs.

EXFOLIATE WISELY

Exfoliation removes dead skin cells, brightens the face, smooths away fine lines, reduces acne scarring, and allows foundation to blend smoothly. For a naturally mild and inexpensive exfoliating treatment, use a half-teaspoon of cornmeal or finely ground almonds applied with your cleanser. Massage in a circular motion for one minute before rinsing. Use once a week for normal to oily skin, every ten days for dry skin.

Microdermabrasion polishes the skin, brings a wonderful glow, and is cost-effective, since you can do it right in your own home. There are many small battery-operated machines on the market for under 30 dollars and you can use your own cleanser with any machine. Use the same schedule as above, once a week, or every ten days if your skin is dry.

The real thing Use only 100% cotton balls (not synthetic cosmetic puffs), Q-tips and washcloths.

A light touch Using your ring finger, apply a small drop (about half the size of a pea) of a line-reducing under-eye cream underneath each eye. Be careful not to overuse the product. Lightly tap and blend across the under-eye area with smooth, soft strokes working towards the nose.

Don't forget Your neck and chest need moisturizer. Work upward on the neck.

Makeup Application

Growing up, Julie never heard anything from her mother about makeup or hair-styling. Her mother had hoped that Julie would figure it out on her own, but Julie didn't have the self-confidence to venture very far past lipstick. The only lesson she ever had was in the girl's bathroom in high school, when one of her friends had said, "Here, try my blue eye shadow." For ten years after that moment, blue eye shadow was still a part of Julie's "getting ready to go out" routine.

As a grown woman Julie had a lovely daughter, Chelsea, whom she nurtured into an intelligent, caring woman like herself. When it came time for Chelsea to get married, Julie was great at preparing for the event but had no idea which direction to steer her daughter regarding makeup, hairstyle, or feeling put together on her big day. Chelsea took the bull by the horns and contacted me to set up an appointment for a face design not only for herself but for her mother as well. They were enthusiastic students and very interested. We reviewed their skin care, choosing appropriate colors, tools, blending techniques, evening wear and what cosmetics they needed to purchase — all while keeping the routine simple. I wanted them to feel beautiful, not just on the wedding day but every day. Julie was having a blast and kept saying, with childlike surprise, "I had no idea!"

Julie and Chelsea left that day armed with a new perspective — they realized they had the power to bring all the elements together and create their own beauty. They also learned how they could take it up a notch and feel glamorous if they wanted. This knowledge, along with a few simple makeup skills, became personal power for Julie. Chelsea had a very good sense of her own style and learned quickly, but was mostly inspired by the change she saw in her mother. She promised herself that she would never feel like an outsider, as her mother had for so many years. They were one of the most beautiful wedding day mother-daughter teams I have ever seen. Julie is a new woman and has never looked better. She smiles more, is more active and feels better now — simply from learning a few things about makeup and her own face. She has said to me repeatedly, "I really like the way I look now. I wish I had done that years ago."

A Favorite Trade Secret

Remove the pad or brush from the base of your home-microdermabrasion machine and, WITHOUT using the exfoliation cream, work the machine in upward, outward circular motions along the cheekbones, cheeks, chin, upper lip and forehead. No product is necessary. The vibrating action of the machine brings blood supply to the surface of your face, boosts collagen production and heals and repairs the skin. This helps get rid of puffy eyes (even though you are not placing it over your eyes) and perks up sagging skin. It is a wonderfully relaxing treatment that brings a youthful glow to the skin, and you can do it anytime — wet or dry, and as often as you like. Just after washing is an easy time to remember. It is a great way to revive or "wake up" a tired face. Working long hours on a set can be tiresome for actors, and this is a powerful tip for those early-morning call times and a great way for you to prevent puffiness and sagging from ever showing up in the first place.

Faces change through the years. Coloring, facial shape, skin texture, and tone all fluctuate just as the styles do, so it's up to us to take our own inventory and stay on top of the changing needs of our face. As cosmetics change, so do the applicators; therefore, we have to stay adaptable at working with new products. What was working for you a few years ago may not be what you need now. Your makeup routine needs to be simple, so knowing what not to do is just as important as knowing what to do.

Here again, I will respond to **the most common grooming mistakes** made by women with specific tips on looking flawless, striking, and beautiful. You CAN figure this out. YOU are your own makeup artist and you can make adjustments that will create star-powered appearance. We've gone over your brows — that's the big first step — so here are the other considerations. Rather than look at yourself and the flaws you are always drawn to first, look with new eyes that really see this process and expect a gorgeous outcome.

KNOW YOUR COLOR TYPE

and you'll take the guess work out of choosing makeup colors.

- If you have blue eyes, pink tones in the palms of your hands, and ash blonde or cool brunette tones in the roots of your hair, then you are a cool-tone person who looks great in pinks, blues, grays, and browns from the cooler end of the spectrum.

- If you tan easily and have green, warm brown, or hazel eyes, with gold or honey high or low lights in your hair, you are a warm-tone person who looks great in soft browns, caramel, canteloupe, and shades of green, to give you an idea.
- Watch what happens when you apply a lip or cheek color. If your skin seems to smooth out and your eye color gets brighter or clearer, the color you have chosen is in your palette and works beautifully. If you look a little tired or blotchy, or suddenly a pimple becomes more noticeable, then the color is too cool for you. Let go of old ideas and inhibitions, step back and see with objective eyes, and feel how it looks on you.

THE FOUNDATION OF ALL MAKEUP is your foundation, and you can make it look as good as a pro. Before blending foundation into your skin, apply one small dot to forehead, nose, upper lip, chin, and cheeks. Then begin blending, using your fingers or a wide foundation brush, being careful not to miss the often overlooked crease under your nostrils. Go from the inside corners of your nose, between your eyes, up to lower lash edge, the lip edge, and along the jaw line. Then pat gently all over to even out and boost circulation.

BLEND CAREFULLY, then check again around the jaw line, out to the hairline, between the eyes at the upper ridge of your nose and around the mouth. Smooth foundation carefully rather than swiping or smearing it around. Softly pat all around to even the finish. This stippling technique will create a smooth, flawless finish as it brings circulation to the face. This stimulates collagen production each time you blend your foundation.

HAVE THE PROPER BRUSH for each cosmetic you wear. Your powder brush does NOT double as a blush brush, or you will continually be moving blush around your face and powder where you need blush. Use a separate natural-bristle brush for each.

REMOVE YOUR MASCARA completely before reapplying or it will clump. Each clump of mascara will get bigger and clumpier with each new coat of mascara that goes over it.

DEFINE YOUR LIPS with lip color from a brush or a lip liner. As time goes by, lip edges fade, and applying a clear gloss over a faded edge still leaves an undefined mouth. Use a neutral color to sharpen up the lip edges, and finish with a cream color or gloss if you want. The important thing is to bring crisp lines to the mouth first.

GET AWAY FROM OLD HABITS that have kept you in a rut because it's all you know. See with different eyes and appreciate your best features. Never apply a cosmetic because someone told you to. Look and know when you've been enhanced. When you can actually see the difference and understand the principles of enhancement, you have become a makeup artist.

Are you staying on track? How are you feeling about your progress in the last few weeks?

_____
_____
_____
_____
_____
_____
_____
_____
_____
_____
_____
_____

This Week's Assignments:

- Read the cosmetic labels in your home and discard the toxic junk.
- Set up your makeup area.
- Wash and moisturize efficiently, adding facial massage as you cleanse.
- Practice face-patting after moisturizer and foundation application.
- Apply eye cream once daily if you're more than 30 years old or if you have dry skin.
- Shape your eyebrows.

Continue To:

- Journal your feelings and experiences. Read over the feelings you journaled about being beautiful.

- Meditate daily.
- Eliminate sugar, white flour, processed foods, milk, and negative thoughts and emotions.
- Practice correct posture at all times.
- Exercise a minimum of four times this week, keeping your sessions up to 75 minutes long. Make sure you allow time for stretching within that time. Challenge yourself by adding an extra half mile to your walk and two sets of additional squats and abdominal exercises.
- Combine food properly.

Today's date _____

> Fitness — if it came in a bottle, everybody would have a great body.
>
> — Cher

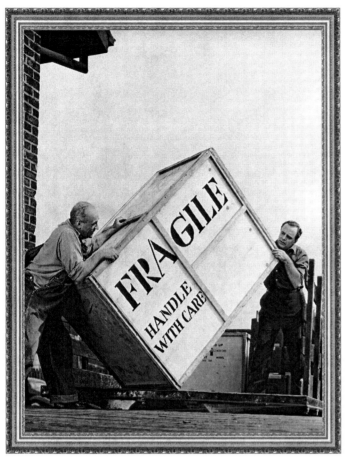

Week 6

This Week's Focus:

Flexibility — Letting Go
Expanding your Exercise Program
Saying You're Sorry
Troubleshooting Hair Problems

Let my People Go!

    Isn't it great to look in the mirror and see a fresher, leaner, more vibrant person looking back? Whether it's smoother skin, a flat tummy, weight loss, more energy, a calmer disposition, or any other change you may have noticed, remember, this is the language of your body speaking as clearly as it can. And it's saying THANKS! You are in Week Six and some changes are expected — your body is leaner, stronger, and more pure. But be mindful of everything happening in your body because there may be some unexpected improvements that surprise you. As time passes and these guidelines become your lifestyle, the positive changes will multiply exponentially. As your body transforms, be sure to notice and rejoice about it. Feel appreciation for a body that can actually improve with use. No other appliance in your home does, but your body gets better as you move and use it. It's a blessing to have a machine that can tone and renew itself without you even thinking about it. You CAN not only feel better but look better in every way. Sit back and enjoy all that happens — and continue to journal about it.

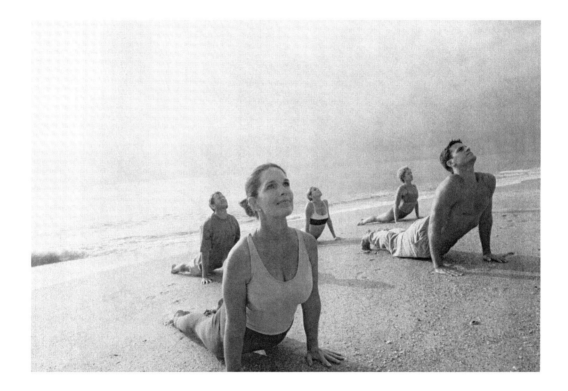

You are an amazingly complex system of energy and intelligence, renewing and opening up to new possibilities for beauty in your body and in your life. Now you can see and feel it happening to you. What a blessing it is to be free, not bound by your old habits. You can now allow the "Authentic You" to make choices.

Deepak Chopra points out that our habits keep us connected to our old inner programming. Once we've let go of old programming, the bondage of the old habit is released. The old habits simply don't serve a purpose any more and will fade away. This may happen effortlessly, or you may occassionally have to use your personal power to make the right choice. But feelings of confidence about your body, and knowing you are worth whatever it takes to be truly healthy and beautiful, will confirm to you that it's all worth it. You will also have a deepened connection to yourself and others. You'll be in touch with your internal wisdom or intuition, with a greater ability to focus. Enjoy all of the positive changes that are happening as the "Authentic You" emerges.

What changes have you have made since Week One that have now become easier?

_____
_____
_____
_____

> *We wear on our faces*
> *the results of what we*
> *believe and how we behave.*
> *— Gordon B. Hinckley*

A Little at a Time

It's with small steps that we are able to make big changes. If you have times you feel you are not "rising to the occasion" or making big enough strides in this process, keep in mind, this is a process. You are on the path. And on every path there are hills and valleys. We are looking for a trend or long-term overall improvement, so don't be hard on yourself, you can still reach your goals. Take a mental trip inside your body and "see" all that it is and all that it does — it's truly a miracle. Having respect for your "machine" will spawn the desire to detoxify and ultimately help you create the body you want to have. Hold on to the intention to have a pure and clean system. Then, break the day into thirds — morning (before noon), afternoon (from noon until four o'clock), and evening (from four until bedtime). Within each portion of the day there will be a meal and some choices. Just for THAT part of the day, be good to yourself and stay on track. As you are aware of each "third" of the day, it's easier to make the choice to eat right — just for that part of the day. You might say no to a processed or junk food that is offered. Or, add some fresh juice or a piece of fruit, or get some exercise. Then feel success when you've been on track for that part of the day.

The morning is the most important "third." The demands of our bodies are highest and it also sets the tone for the rest of the day. If your morning has gone by and you are on track — great! It's downhill from there. If you've hit a bump in the road, take it one step at a time. It becomes easier and you'll feel less pressured. If you can take some of the pressure of failure off of yourself, you are more likely to transition into the fit person you'd like to be.

Letting Go — What are You Still Packing Around?

In my career, I have been on location in many countries and states and in every kind of weather or type of place you can imagine. It is hard to name a place where somebody hasn't set up a camera and crew and started shooting. I will always be grateful for the many years of adventure.

Years ago, I was on location shooting a film in a convalescent facility. There was a lighting problem on set, and I knew there was going to be a long break while they re-lit. I went to the front desk and asked who the oldest person in the facility was, and if I could go and visit them. Her name was Anna, and she was 97. I went to see her and was impressed with how alert she was. She was happy to have a visitor and had lots to say. It was wonderful to hear her speak about a long life so objectively. As she spoke of her life, I noticed something remarkable about her. Although she had suffered many losses and trials, she did not harbor regrets or sadness because of the bad things that had happened to her. Instead, she spoke objectively about them. It was clear she had let go of sadness and regret. After almost a century, Anna still lived a life open to possibilities with a loving spirit. This set the tone in her body for continuous healing and longevity. Her ability to let go is a trait common among perky, spirited seniors that have outlived their peers. In our own quest for longevity and good health, we must internalize flexibility and an attitude of "letting go."

Obviously we can't control the outcome of every situation. Being flexible means releasing ourselves from attachments and from our desire for control.

Holding onto ideas and being rigid about how we think things should be brings stress to the body and speeds up the aging process. Flexibility means being open to new possibilities and being willing to embrace the unknown, where all new potential lies.

This doesn't mean letting go of your goals. They direct your life in the path it will go. Flexibility requires letting go of your attachment to how you think things SHOULD be. Thinking "I should have this position" or "I should make more money" only brings a sense of being unfulfilled or not having what you want. Happiness comes from knowing that whatever the outcome, you will be able to embrace the unknown with curiosity and a willingness to progress. Many people spend an entire lifetime trying to find security through their attachments —"he who dies with the most toys wins." Things do not bring happiness. They are about the past. Flexibility looks to the future and is progressive. Being flexible, not only in your body but also in your mind, brings a disposition to the body where health can thrive.

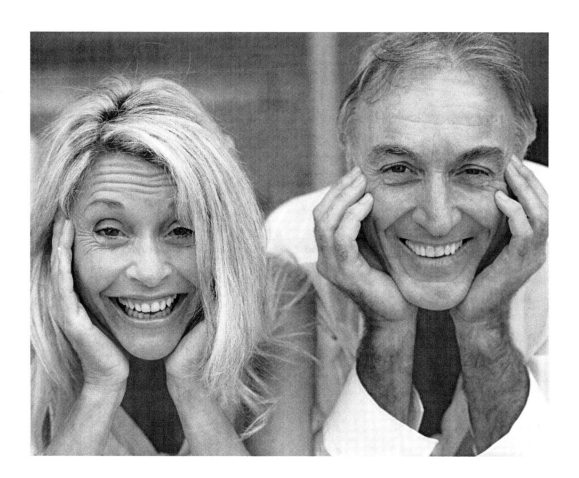

Adding on

Add these postures to your workout to improve your flexibility and gain strength. Allow physical flexibility to translate into mental flexibility. These exercises are in sequence. When added to the warm-up you learned in Week Four, this becomes a smooth, efficient, body-sculpting exercise routine. Focus on your body and breath, let it clear your mind as it shapes your body. Set aside time for at least four exercise sessions this week.

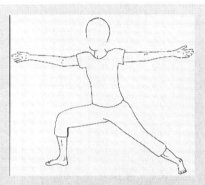

Widen your stance with the toes on your right foot turned to the right. As you lunge into the quad on the right side, look down and check to make sure your kneecap is directly above your heel. Make sure your thigh is parallel to the floor and your knee is not hyper-extended. Extend the arms straight out, lengthening from fingertip to fingertip, with your shoulders relaxed and your hands soft. Breath from your belly. Hold here for a few breaths.

With your stance still wide and your toes turned out, breathe in. As you exhale, lunge into the quad on the right side. Set your right forearm on your right thigh. Keep your chest facing forward, left arm straight and extended so it is up by your ear. Press through the side of your left foot — making sure your left pinkie toes are pressed into the floor — and drop your hips toward the floor. Make sure your shoulders are stacked so you don't bend forward. Lengthen up through your hand. Look up through your fingers and breathe. Hold for 10 counts. Lower your arm and use the quad to press back up. Repeat on the other side.

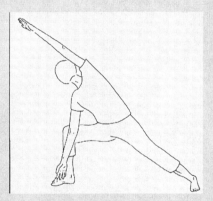

Week 6   149

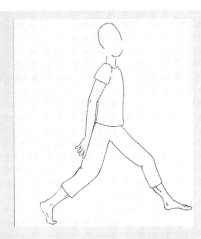

Push back to neutral, still in a wide stance, and turn your ribs in the same direction as your toes and hips. Let the heel behind you come off the floor. Breathe in.

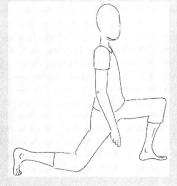

Drop into a lunge as you exhale. Push back and repeat for eight more lunges.

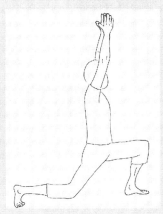

With your stance still wide, turn to your right, pivoting on the toes of your back foot. As your back heel comes up, bring your hips around to the right — bringing yourself into a lunge position. Spread the toes on your front foot and plant that foot into the floor. Your chest should face straight ahead and be aligned with your toes. Lunge down as you count to four and then back up as you count to four. Repeat for a set of six. Before your last lunge, take a deep breath in and raise both arms with your palms facing each other, and hold low in the lunge. Find an eye spot to focus on and stay here for twenty seconds.

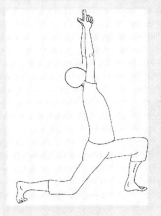

Press your palms together, interlace your fingers, release your index fingers, and relax your head and neck as you arch back. Let your eyes follow your fingers. Hold here for a few breaths. Let your hands float apart, and use your quads to press back to neutral.

Healing by Saying you're Sorry

Forgiveness is intimately linked to the healing process, and even though it may be the most difficult step in the process for some, it is what truly frees us. The postures above address your physical flexibility. But equally important are your mental and emotional flexibility. With forgiveness, we let go and gain flexibility.

Resentment and grudges held inside of you hide your radiance and beauty. They cause you more damage than the person they're aimed at and require energy to maintain. This deficit of healing energy ages the body. Bitterness is toxic and, when held onto for years, is easy to recognize as sternness even when the face is relaxed. It causes the face to appear less vital and bright. Bitterness creates a lifeless or grim face more prone to wrinkling. In order for your body to have 100% of its healing capacity, this blocked energy must be allowed to flow.

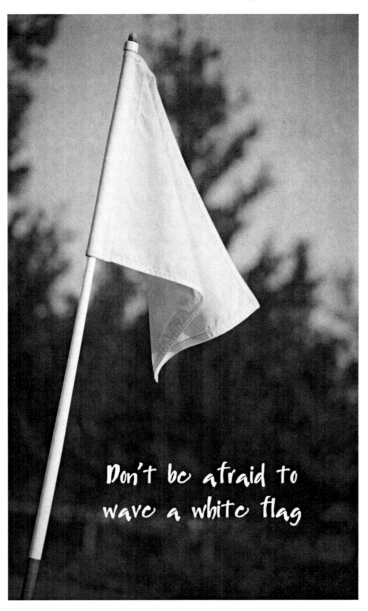

Don't be afraid to wave a white flag

Since we are imperfect, we have all been hurt by someone else and we have all wronged someone else. Through meditation and the lifestyle adjustments you have made in the past few weeks, you are now focused on positive aspects of your life. The time is right to take the opportunity to make amends so complete healing can take place within your heart and body and allow your authentic beauty to shine through. If a hurt or a strained relationship exists in your life, take the steps to make right your part.

List here those you need to forgive. Make a separate list of those who you need to make amends with.

_____
_____
_____
_____
_____
_____
_____
_____

Feel into your heart area as you make the lists. Have the intention to let go of any pain or discomfort that you feel in this area. Listen to your body and what it is telling you. Listen to your breath for a moment as you are making your lists. Review the list and allow spaciousness to come into your heart. Stay with this feeling for a few breaths or as long as you like. Feel love from inside of you. Listen to what your intuition is telling you: it is the wisdom of your body mending your soul. Take a deep breath and know that you can let this be.

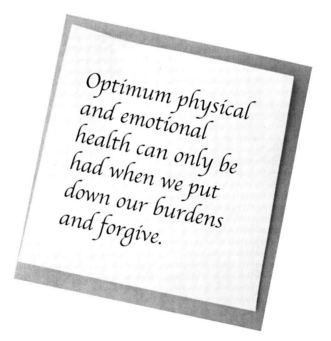

Optimum physical and emotional health can only be had when we put down our burdens and forgive.

To those on your list, you may write a letter, speak to them in person, or have a friend mediate if circumstances require it. Say you are sorry for your part in whatever wrong has taken place. You are the one in charge of your actions, and consequently your health, so you will be the one that will benefit by rising to this occasion. Their response is not what matters. They may not be where you are spiritually or emotionally and may not know how to react. But no matter what their response is, you will be free from carrying the burden and able to reclaim energy and fulfillment.

The Bigger the Hair, the Closer to God

In the 1960s I was a little girl, the seventh of eight children. Four of these children were older sisters. They were beautiful and went to lots of parties and on many dates. The big beehive hairdo was all the rage then. I sat on the laundry hamper with my face in my hands for hours just to watch it all happen. I remember those hairdos so clearly. It was a fine art to get it teased up just right. They were fabulous brunettes, and I thought they were stunning. It was my job, as per an agreement that my mother didn't know about, to wait up for my two oldest sisters and brush the "rats" (as we used to call them) out of their big-beehive, teased-up hairdos. As they sat on the couch I would sit behind them on the back of the couch and carefully and tediously brush out all the tangles. For this I was paid usually a nickel or a half stick of gum (on a good day it would be a whole stick of gum). I learned then that grooming is an important ritual full of ceremony that lifts the spirit.

No matter what era you grew up in, there will be styling techniques you learn — and some you skip over — because of what fashion dictates. No matter what the current styles are, you are the one in charge of your 'do. You will need the skills to change with the times. So, whether or not you are good at managing a big beehive, all that matters now is whether or not you are open to new grooming techniques and styles.

Back to the Beginning

Do this little test — Grab a section of hair on the top of your head, hold it tightly and move it back and forth. Is the hair firmly stuck in place or does the scalp move as you move your hand back and forth? Your scalp should be loose and move about an inch in each direction. To maintain a healthy head of hair, the circulation under your scalp must flow; the scalp should be pliable and move with the hair. Scalp massage is an important part of shampooing. In all the workshops and private consultations I have done over the years, it's been mind-boggling to find so many grown-ups that have not learned the technique of a proper shampoo. Let's start with the basics (even if you are a grown-up, let's go over this just

Shampooing — Are we really going over this? Yes, we are. The first part of your body to wash in the shower or bath is your hair — this allows time for your conditioner to stay on the ends of your hair while you finish bathing. Wet hair first, then put a quarter-sized amount of shampoo into the palm of your hand. Use both hands to distribute the shampoo to the roots and scalp of the hair only. Never apply shampoo to the ends of your hair. Shampoo is drying to the already dead part of your hair. The rinsing action provides enough cleansing to the ends of the hair. Remember the base of the neck, above the ears and under the thick section on the crown. Use the pads of your fingers and massage slowly in a circular motion, for one minute — going over the entire head.

Take some deep breaths, moving the scalp to increase circulation. Do not use your fingernails on your scalp. Nail scratching can irritate the scalp and wet hair can cause hang nails and split nails. Rinse thoroughly and repeat as many times as necessary depending on the thickness of your hair.

Protect the investment of time and money that you have spent on your hair by using the proper type of shampoo. If you have color-treated hair, make sure you are using a shampoo for color-treated hair. If your hair is thick and shoulder length or longer, you should wash your hair in a different position every third or fourth shampoo. For example, if you normally wash your hair in the shower with your head tipped back, you need to bend your head over a sink and wash with your hair falling forward as well. This allows you to thoroughly clean all areas of your scalp, get in between hard-to-reach hair follicles, and make your hair smell fresher!

Tip

Hold your hair brush in your hand. With your thumb, press on the bristles and move back and forth. The bristles should be flexible and move easily so it will "give" as it glides through your hair. The bristles should not be sharp. There should be a small ball tip to massage the scalp as you brush. Never use a brush with metal or hard plastic bristles. They are too stiff and will damage, split, or break hair.

Conditioning — Squeeze excess water out of the hair, put conditioner into the palm of one hand — about the size of a quarter. Use both hands to distribute conditioner to the ends of your hair, being careful to not get it too close to the scalp. The roots of your hair have natural oils from your scalp and do not need to be conditioned. Unnecessarily conditioning the scalp can cause hair to look greasy and feel limp and lifeless. Massage conditioner into the ends only and leave on your hair for several minutes as you finish your bath. Rinse thoroughly. Ultra-fine hair and even some short styles need to skip the conditioning step to achieve the desired fullness.

Styling — Your hair should move and shine with a style that reflects your personality and lets you feel like you. Here are some clues that your current hairstyle may not be best for you:
- Your style takes too much time (more than 25 minutes).
- You feel you can't style it to your liking, so you often just let it go or pull it back in clips or a ponytail.
- You are using the same styling products and tools that you have used for more than five or ten years.
- It no longer makes the most of your best features.

From the following, make a list of what you really like about your hair. This will be List A:

_____
_____
_____
_____
_____
_____

Then make another list of what makes your hair hard for you to work with.

low hairline • high forehead • limp • fine • thick • curly • straight • shiny • dull • dry • good color • coarse • frizzy • uneven curl • easy to curl • has body • damaged • over-processed • brittle • chemically treated • in good shape • doesn't hold curl

This will be List B:

_____
_____

Now list the hair products you are currently using:

_____
_____

Compare the products to List B. These products should address the bad features of your hair, while enhancing the features on List A. For example, if your hair is thin and fine, you should be using products like volumizing mousse, fine mist thickening hair spray or a root lifter. If you love the shiny quality of your hair you should not be using a heavy lacquer hairspray. Consider your styling technique as you look at these lists. If List B says your curl is uneven or your hair is frizzy, you should have a ceramic flat iron and an anti-frizz product to correct these. If your forehead is low, bangs may not be a good option. You are the hairdresser, so take a moment and decide if your choices are optimal.

Shopping list — List here products and styling tools you need to work with your hair type.

_____
_____
_____
_____
_____
_____
_____
_____

Simply Sleep

Your rest is so important right now — be in bed at 9:30! Never go to bed with food in your stomach; feel your digestion process and know when your stomach has emptied. Sleeping right after eating will bring weight gain and a slower metabolism.

What a path you have traveled in the last six weeks! Heartfelt congratulations. There has been soul-searching and serious dedication and commitment on your part to achieve the internal cleansing and bring you this far.

Are you Still Craving Sugar?

For another reminder about eating healthy and clearing your system, let's talk about sugar. In case you're still having a hard time letting go — here are a few more reasons to get sugar and sweets out of your life. [1, 2, 3, 4, 5, 6, 7]

Sugar

- disturbs the mineral relationship in the body
- causes cravings, which brings weight gain
- IS AN ADDICTIVE SUBSTANCE
- causes tooth decay and periodontal disease
- weakens eyesight and can cause myopia and cataracts
- disrupts hormone balance
- promotes emotional outbursts
- can cause gallstones and appendicitis
- increases the risk of Crohn's disease, alcoholism and ulcerative colitis
- CAUSES IRRITABILITY, HYPERACTIVITY, LACK OF FOCUS, AND ANXIETY IN CHILDREN
- promotes gas by feeding colon bacteria
- raises cholesterol
- causes inflammation, which reduces immune response
- reduces insulin sensitivity
- contributes to Alzheimer's disease
- decreases growth hormone
- increases delta, alpha and theta brain waves
- BRINGS CHROMIUM AND COPPER DEFICIENCY

---

1. Flaws, Bob. The Tao of Healthy Eating, Redwing Books, 2008.
2. Ni, Maoshing, Dr. Secrets of Self Healing, Penguin Group, 2008
3. Ceriello, A. Oxidative Stress Glycemic Regulation, Metabolism. Feb 2000
4. Perricone, Nicholas, M.D. The Wrinkle Cure, Rodale Inc., Warner Books, 2001.
5. Roizen, M.D., Michael F., Oz, M.D. Frank. You On A Diet, New York: Free Press, 2006.
6. "Four Habits That Weaken the Immune System." Immune Central. www.immunecentral.com/templates/info_template.cfm/1696/70/1
7. Appleton, Nancy. Lick the Sugar Habit, New York: Avery Penguin Putnam, 1988.

Sugar

prevents absorption of magnesium and calcium

PROMOTES WRINKLES

weakens the spleen

increases belly fat

contributes to diabetes, heart disease, and osteoporosis

leaves you more prone to infectious disease

suppresses the immune system

causes hypoglycemia

causes arthritis and asthma

can cause premature aging

feeds cancer

wreaks havoc with PMS

desensitizes the hypothalamus

reduces high density lipoproteins

adds bulk to the body

reduces natural defense against bacterial infection

PROMOTES FAT STORAGE

raises triglycerides

CAUSES DAMAGING CHANGES IN THE KIDNEYS

lowers the amount of vitamin E in the bloodstream

creates an acidic condition in the digestive tract

This Week's Assignments:

- Continue to eat foods in proper combination.
- Meditate daily.
- Add the new exercises from this Week to the warm-up you learned in Week 4 for a smooth, fluid routine.
- Practice making the complete routine flow. Beginning with the complete routine, work out a minimum of four times this week. Add the routine to your walking or other workout to total 60–75 minutes.
- Use your list of names and make amends.
- Purchase the products and styling tools that you identified to be the best for your hair.
- Maintain eyebrows, using a brow pencil daily if necessary.
- Be mindful of your water intake this week. Be sure to stay hydrated.

Today's date _____

At 50 you get the face you deserve.

— Coco Chanel

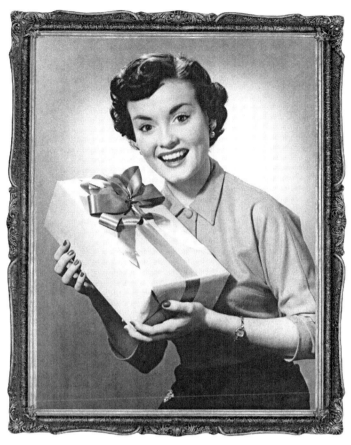

Week 7

This Week's Focus:

Your Face: Now is the Time to be Beautiful
Managing Stress
Posture Maintenance
Five Stars a Day
Dealing and Healing

Rise and Shine
From my column "All Health's Breaking Loose"

My favorite outdoor event of the year arrives in early spring: sweet peas begin blooming in my backyard. Their miracle is knowing when to pop up and when to lie sleeping. The earth is a system of cyclical miracles of which we are a part, and the intelligence of our bodies relies on it. Night follows day, and restful sleep replenishes our energy and spirit. We arise to a new beginning and get another chance to take charge of our health.

Your body loves morning. Whether you're heavy-handed on the snooze button or "Miss Perky Pants," you'll look and feel your best after an a.m. grooming routine. It only takes a few minutes to nourish your body and soul, and once that's done your mind is better prepared to handle anything that may come your way. Here are a few tips to choose from to help you design your own morning ritual:

- Walk straight to the kitchen and prepare a refreshing cup of herbal tea with honey and lemon. Let it cool slightly, and sip it as you prepare for the day.
- Use a scraper or toothbrush to remove accumulated bacteria from the back of your tongue for fresher breath.
- Eat fruit before anything else so your digestive cycle starts with fiber.
- Light your metabolic fire with exercise. Every system of your body will function better throughout the day with the added oxygen, and you'll continue to burn extra calories throughout the day.

We arise to a new beginning and get another chance to take charge of our health

- Set your posture standard. Lift your ribs; then with both hands, reach behind your back, interlace your fingers, palms pressed together if you can, and straighten your arms to open up your chest. Hold for a few seconds.
- During your shower, brush your skin all over with a natural bristle brush, working towards the heart. Exfoliating and invigorating the skin is a wake-up call to your whole body.
- Take a cold rinse at the end of your shower to close pores (protecting your immune system) and hair follicles (for shiny hair).
- Pat your face lightly for one minute after applying moisturizer or shaving. This mini-facial treatment renews collagen, plumps up lines and wrinkles, and brings circulation and a radiant glow to the face.
- Take three slow, deep breaths, filling your body with all the oxygen it can hold. Bring to mind your gifts and blessings, and then exhale slowly with a smile.

We're intimately connected to the earth's cycles — just like my sweet peas. If we work with those cycles, we can bring a little slice of heaven to each day with a personalized morning grooming routine. Whatever heaven means to you, I hope it smells like sweet peas there. **End of Column**

Tired and Stressed Out?

From my column "All Health's Breaking Loose"

Duke was a family friend — a gentle, average-sized guy with a large family. He and his wife had just purchased a new refrigerator and stocked it with groceries when their house caught fire. After all the kids had gotten out safely, Duke ran back inside and, with his senses heightened, he picked up the new, fully-stocked refrigerator and carried it outside. The next day, after the fire was out and their home was salvaged, it was time to move the fridge back inside. This time it took three strong men to move it.

What Duke experienced was the heightened physical performance that comes from an adrenal function in full swing. With adrenaline coursing through his veins he briefly had the strength of three men. That is the job of your adrenal glands. These two walnut-sized, triangular-shaped organs sit right on top of your kidneys and, as part of your endocrine system, release and regulate hormones, including adrenaline, as needed to deal with the stress you experience[1]. Kind of makes you feel all warm and fuzzy just knowing your body looks after you like that, doesn't it?

We all have times in our lives when our adrenal glands go into action, and yet, we're not even aware of it. For someone who has had an injury, or is suffering a major illness such as cancer, diabetes, or heart disease, stress is suffered on two levels. First, there is the psychological stress or the very idea that this frightening illness or injury has entered your body and your life; second, there is the biological stress, or what the illness is causing on a cellular level.

These small but mighty organs are on constant alert to deal with your stress. But your adrenals don't stop there; they also "have your back" during times of emotional crisis such as divorce, caring for a seriously ailing loved one, the loss of a job, continual overworking, or a death in the family. These amazing tiny organs (weighing about as much as a grape) kick into high gear whenever needed. They are the superheroes of our bodies! The trouble starts when the stress becomes long term. They're sprinters, not long-distance runners. Even though they aren't built for it, they'll keep trying until there is a major strain in the body. You may not even recognize what is happening in your body as "strain." But if you listen, you'll understand the language of your body — IT IS SPEAKING TO YOU. Some of the signs: feeling

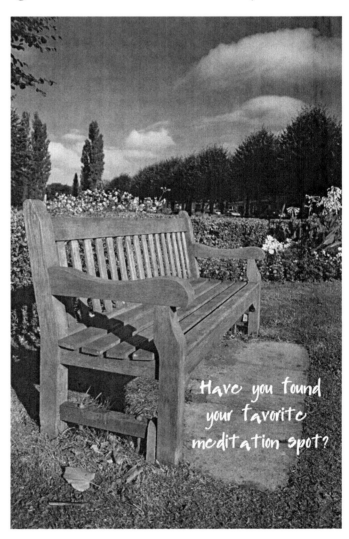

Have you found your favorite meditation spot?

---

1. Marcelle, Pick, OB/GYN, NP. "Eating to Support Your Adrenal Glands." 17 August 2009. www.womentowomen.com/adrenalfatigue/adrenalglandnutrition.aspx

tired for no reason, trouble sleeping, slight depression or just feeling "tapped out," moodiness, lethargy, and using colas, coffee, chocolate, or snack foods to get through the day.

If you have been used to living your life in the fast lane, remember you are the one driving and you are the one who has to slow things down. The fast-lane living of modern times has made adrenal fatigue commonplace, and most people don't even know it exists. But your body knows what it is and if you've experienced some of the above-mentioned symptoms, you may be suffering from adrenal fatigue. It is intimately connected to various ailments including chronic fatigue, fibromyalgia, heightened menopause and PMS symptoms, heart disease, and a host of other "new" illnesses that have doctors in a quandary.

Getting out of the fast lane is easier said than done. We are creatures of habit and when you have been chronically busy for years, finding time to stop is difficult. It feels unproductive somehow. And yet, to stop sawing and sharpen the saw may be the most productive thing you have done in a long time. The stress you feel is only the stress you perceive. To one person the events that cause you to say, "I've had a terrible morning, my life is a mess" may cause another person to smile and simply say, "Oops, sorry I'm late." **End of Column**

Through your meditation practice, we began in Week One to relieve the burden on your adrenal glands and thyroid. At this point, healing has begun to take place. You have given yourself (your adrenals and thyroid glands) a great gift and fortified your long-term health by creating a calmer, more peaceful life.

If your adrenal glands could give you their most important mantra it would be:

Don't sweat the small stuff. And it's all small stuff.

Then:
- Remember to find quiet time to sit and meditate daily, whether you're at the office or home. Release your thoughts and just breathe.
- Go with the ebb and flow. When obligations slow down, prioritize that time and take a morning off here or there, as the season allows, to enjoy some personal time. It doesn't have to be expensive — sit on your patio and sip a cup of tea, or go for a leisurely walk. Walk slowly for a few blocks and breathe while you think thoughts about the goodness in your life.
- Give yourself a facial or other personal treat.

List here one or more inexpensive (or free) personal treats you can do at home that help you feel calm and blessed:

More Ideas for your Personal Treats

- A facial scrub followed by light moisturizer.
- A self foot massage.
- A moment to breathe fresh air by a fountain in your yard.
- Resting for a moment in the sunshine to watch your pet play.
- If you have a lot of reasons to hold tension in your body then you might need help to get the tension out. Get a massage.

Our top priority (since you began this program) has been to release stress from your body. We have practiced through a myriad of techniques and modalities, and even though it may have been challenging at times — it has been oh, so worth it. I'm hoping you are aware of the healing that has taken place in your body. A calmer, more peaceful sensation in your body will confirm to you that it has.

Prevent that "Tapped-Out" Feeling

- Write bigger on your calendar. It leaves less room for your "to-do list."
- Release your worrisome thoughts — just knowing that whatever you might be worrying about will be better off if you are not throwing negative energy after it.
- Think about what you are doing and thinking when you feel positive, light-hearted and happy:
- Pick a spot where you go daily. Each time you are there, take a moment to feel appreciation for all you have. Call this your "appreciation spot" and make it a daily exercise. When you feel lucky and blessed, stress is as far away from you as it can possibly be.

Where is your "appreciation spot"?

_____

_____

Your Face Says It All

If you're **content**, at peace, **TOXIC**, **TIRED**, *prone to depression*, **energetic**, or **healthy** — no matter what — it will show up in your face. Your face can only be honest about your internal processes and how you really feel, emotionally and at a cellular level. The face is a reliable indicator that tells the world how you treat yourself. When we don't listen to our bodies, we are more likely to abuse them — and it all gets written in the face. A close look into anyone's face will tell you …

… If they are eating foods that their body cannot handle (graininess in the skin, puffiness, blotchiness, or discoloration).
… If they are unable to sleep well (sagging, lifeless eyes, under-eye circles, chalky skin).
… If they have had long-term depression or stress (fine crepiness to the skin, rapid aging).
… If they don't get enough exercise (dry, chalky skin, lack of tone, fluid retention).
… If they smoke (dry, chalky skin, upper lip wrinkles, poor texture, a stagnant appearance to the skin, lack of smoothness and shine).
… If they have a tendency for anger (forehead tension and furrowed brow lines).
… If they over-drink (puffiness around the nose and cheeks, swollen appearance to the skin, broken capillaries).
… If they overeat (a swollen or struggling appearance to the skin).

BUT if they're generally happy and content (glowing skin, a fine texture, smooth skin quality, young-looking skin).

AND if they're eating a super foods diet — you can't hide the brightness and smooth quality in the skin texture!

This week's goal is to learn about your face, recognize any facial changes, decide precisely which tools you need, and acquire the skills necessary to create a smooth, toned, vibrant face. For women, we'll develop a professional make-up finish and for men a well-groomed, flattering appearance. During the 30 years I've groomed celebrities for appearances, I've often been asked, "How did you get her face to look so smooth? She was stunning, what's the secret?" Or, "Is he really that good-looking up close?" If an actor is prone to skin problems and lacking perfect features, it is still possible for them to look stunning on the red carpet if the right care is taken and specific products applied with the appropriate tools.

For Women

Before we even begin to talk about applying makeup, first things first. Let's talk about your tools — applicators, brushes, sponges, and miscellaneous.

Good makeup tools are an investment in yourself. They allow proper usage of your cosmetics. Cheap or bad brushes do more harm than good. The little plastic brush that manufacturers include inside compacts should go right into the garbage or be given to your kids for their art work — just don't use it on your face. If cost is an issue, shop for one brush at a time until you have a completely personalized set. Good brushes last for years and meanwhile, you will recoup the cost and have a more professional representation of yourself. Look for brushes with natural fiber bristles, such as sable, mink or goat hair. The handle should be easy to grip and not too long, so it is easy to keep in your drawer and touch-up bag. Purchase only the brushes you need. Get rid of old brushes or brushes that may have come with a set if you are not using them. They clutter up your space. Keep it simple.

Once you know the makeup routine that is optimum for you, choose from the list below to assemble a collection of tools that will streamline your application.

Decide Which of these Brushes you Need

Two stars mark the "must haves":

Foundation brush to apply a perfectly smooth foundation. Gives better coverage with the same amount of liquid makeup. A sponge is fine too, but uses up foundation faster.

Eyeshadow brush allows perfect blending and control. Creates a smoother, cleaner finish than sponge tip applicators.

Fine-tip eye de liner for under-eye shadow effects, such as brushed on eyeliner.

A rouge brush to apply powder, dry cheek color, bronzer, or to blend over your eyeshadow. Use in a sweeping motion — do not jam bristles into the face. This is a good basic and can be washed with mild soap. Gently shake excess water out, smooth hairs back into place, wrap with a folded tissue to hold the bristles in place, and allow to air dry.

Tweezers: A must for anyone who has eyebrows.

*A good quality **latex sponge** to blend all types of foundation. Also can be used for blending eyeshadow. These are disposable, but if washed occasionally with a mild soap they can last for weeks. Keep them on hand and replace as needed. Use sharp scissors to trim the sharp angle from the edges.

*A **lip brush** to apply lip color and gloss. If you have cracking in your upper or lower lip, this one is a must. The tiny hairs in the brush deposit the lip color right down into the cracks, filling in the tiny crevices of the mouth — unlike a sponge tip gloss applicator that will glide across the surface and cause smearing and running. If your life is filled with long days and not much time for touch-ups, your lip color will last longer when applied with a brush.

*An **angle tip brush** or small precision brush will create a "smoky" look when applying eyeshadow to the under-eye area. Without an angle tip on the brush, you could end up with too much shadow, making you look tired instead of "smoky." This brush is also used for applying and blending shadows to the lower eyelid, creating a soft, smooth look instead of a "drawn on" look.

*A **powder puff** can be used if you plan to attend an event and need to keep your makeup application perfect over a very long period of time. But use powder sparingly and with caution. Overuse of powder causes skin to appear dry and lifeless. If you have acne scars or rough skin, a puff may be helpful to achieve more coverage with your foundation base.

*An **eyebrow brush** is necessary for brows that are curly, long, thick or unruly. Brows can be trained by using your eyebrow brush regularly.

List here the tools you need to add or replace. Add them to your kit as soon as possible.

_____
_____
_____
_____
_____
_____
_____
_____
_____
_____
_____
_____

Prepping the Skin

Begin with a clean face. Lightly dot your daytime moisturizer onto the cheek bones, chin, upper lip, forehead and neck (three dots on the neck). Blend carefully, directing the strokes upward on your neck, gently outward towards the cheek bones, and across the upper lip and forehead. Take a deep breath as your fingers glide across your skin. Visualize a smooth surface, and pause on a wrinkle, blemish or scar that concerns you. With your fingers placed gently over the trouble spot, lightly massage in a small, circular motion. Breathe in and visualize your face completely smooth. Release any tension in your face and exhale.

Use a small amount (about half the size of a pea) of eye cream on your ring finger and blend toward the nose. Finish by patting with light, rapid, open-hand taps all over the face, moving to every place you applied moisturizer. Patting brings circulation to the skin, and revives it. The moisturizer application and cleansing breath work takes approximately one minute. Let your face rest for a few minutes as you continue your morning routine. Now your foundation will glide beautifully over a smooth surface.

Foundation Application

Dot your foundation on the forehead, the nose, on the cheekbones, the jaw, and chin. For daytime wear, you may disregard the neck and, using a foundation brush or your fingers, blend to a light finish. For a photo or special event, you will need to blend down as your wardrobe neck line requires. Blend gently, without rubbing. Keep in mind that as you look in the mirror, the three-dimensional surface of your face has become a flat reflection. Often forgotten are the following areas:

- The delicate areas on the inside of the nose up between the eyes.
- Around the corners of the nostrils.
- From the cheekbones out to the hairline.
- Around the mouth.

Consider what you are trying to accomplish, as if you had been hired to take care of YOUR face. Years of "quickly dabbing here and there" is a difficult habit to break — but we are striving for a flawless finish.

Facial Highlighting

Before highlighting, reduce any visible redness. Most problems in your skin will have a reddish cast to them, such as acne, small broken capillaries, and scars. To counteract the reddish cast, you will need a concealer product lighter than your foundation that has a slight yellow tone (yellow neutralizes red). Whether you are working with a pencil with flesh tone lead, a pot of concealer with a fine-tip brush or a highlighter with a brush-tip applicator that has product already inside the tube, you can achieve the same effect. There are usually only two or three shades of concealer in either of these options to choose from. Test the colors on your skin. Apply a small dot in the center of the problem area and blend outward until it is no longer visible.

This technique will brighten the face and take years off your age; it is a valuable trick and can be done quickly and easily after you apply foundation. Or, on a busy morning running quick errands, you can skip the foundation and use only this step followed by a little bronzer to smooth out the skin tone.

In a room with natural light, stand about 18 inches away from a large mirror and look directly at your face. What lines, wrinkles or bone structure imperfections do you notice? You notice them because of the shadow they create. The valley or "ditch" created by the wrinkle is shadowed and can't receive light and thus you see a wrinkle. A nose that is too short needs a highlight to lengthen it, while a nose that is too long creates a shadow on the upper lip that may need to be lightened as well. When eyelids become puffy, they hang just enough to create a tiny little shadow on the outside corner of the eye. Look for any shadows, discoloration or dark spots. Don't be overcritical and attempt to change everything you see. Every face has a natural topography that is beautiful.

Dab your brush into the highlighter, then, on the back of your hand or a clean surface, bring the loaded brush to a fine point. If you are using a pencil, make sure the lead is fresh. Check these areas for lines and shadows, highlighting only the ones that apply to your face:
- under the eyes
- in the center of the forehead
- under the outside corners of the eyes
- the nasolabial folds that run from the nose to the sides of the mouth
- the horizontal line below your lower lip and just above your chin

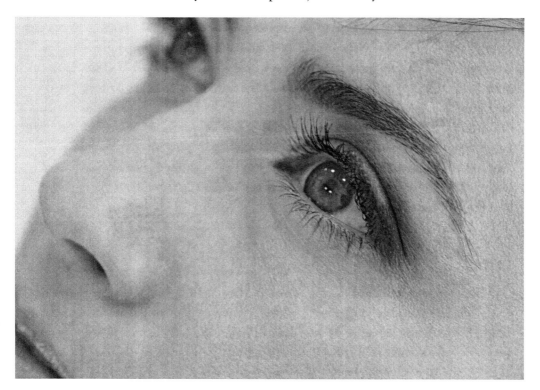

Decide what you need, and gently draw a thin line down in the crevice or shadow and blend the edges. Be careful not to wipe the line off completely and don't let it remain a visible "line," but blend it carefully. As in the principles of art, LIGHT throws forward, and DARK throws back. So, by strategically placing highlights where you need them, you are erasing wrinkles and brightening your face. Just as your other lifestyle adjustments have made your body look and feel younger, this technique takes years off your face!

Cheek Color

To create a perfectly smooth finish to your base you will need to continue to work with cream-based products. Using a cream rouge or cream bronzer that is soft and muted, blend carefully across the sun zone or the places the sun hits your face naturally, as in nose, cheekbones and forehead. If your skin is smooth and ceramic-looking, it is all right to have a little iridescence to your rouge. If you have problem or aging skin, sparkle or sheen intensifies flaws, so stay with a matte color. Look in the mirror. Is your face narrow, wide or oval? If your face is narrow, there will not be much space from the sides of your nose to the hairline in front of your ear. If your face is wide, there will be more space or width from your nose out to this hairline. The goal is to create the appearance of an oval face and bring your features into balance with the shape of your face. Rouge placement is capable of bringing balance to an imperfect shape of face. Using a latex sponge lightly tapped into your cheek color, blend outward toward the temples, along the cheekbone. If you have a narrow face, make sure not to come in too close to your nose. Keeping the color out towards the hairline will create a more "oval" appearance. If you have a full or wide face, you will blend along the cheekbone and bring your cheek color in towards the center of your face, and then blend the edges softly downward. This will minimize the fleshy area on the front of your face, creating a more oval appearance. If you have a double chin or heavy neck, use your matte bronzer to lightly blend down under the jaw line to "slim down" and create a more boned jaw area.

Powder

Powder is wonderful for setting makeup that has to hold for a long period of time, whether you're having photos taken or attending an all-day event without time for touch-ups. Because of hot camera lights and long hours, powder works great for television also. But for daywear, a fresh, dewy look to the face and a light feeling to makeup is best. Use powder if you are having a photo taken, as it reflects light and will give you a smoother look and reduce shine to the camera eye. Or if you have troubled skin or your job requires you to look good for many

Tip

Your large powder brush should never be used for cheek color. Keep it away from colored powders or you will be adding rouge color all over your face as you blend your powder. Do not push the brush into the skin; instead, gently glide it across using the side of the bristles so they don't break..

Week 7   171

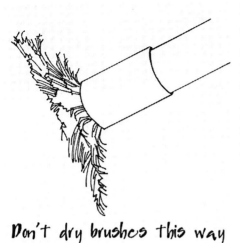

Don't dry brushes this way

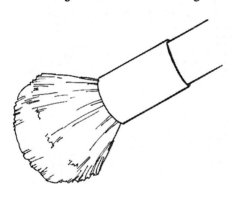

Dry them this way

hours at a time, use it as you feel the need and keep it with you for touch-ups. YOU are your own makeup artist and YOU will have to decide how often you use powder. To keep your makeup colors truer, a yellow tone or translucent powder will set makeup without being visible on the skin. If you have problem skin with a ruddy, red tone, use a powder with a yellow tone.

Tap a large powder brush into translucent powder and shake gently so the brush is loaded lightly, or glide across pressed powder until brush is loaded. Stroke across the face to distribute evenly, brushing across a few times. Be sure to lightly powder your eyelids so your shadow will blend smoothly. This creates a powder finish to the surface of the skin. If you want to "punch up" your cheek color, you may now use your powder cheek color lightly at the upper edge of your cheekbone. If you want a "sunny" tanned look, you may dust lightly with a powdered bronzer at the upper edge of the cheek bones and lightly in the T-zone to warm up the face. Pressed powder is less messy and great to take along in your bag. It is the same product as loose powder and often is preferred because it keeps things simple. In any case, use powder sparingly.

Eyeshadow

Now that there is an even powder finish to your face and eyelids, your eyeshadow will glide on smoothly and blend easily. If you did not use powder on your face, the eyelids will need to be prepped for shadow; otherwise, you will not be able to blend your eyeshadow smoothly. This is easy and I don't want you to think of it as an extra step if you are not used to doing it. To keep it simple, select a powdered eyeshadow trio that has one light, neutral color such as beige, ivory

> ### Tip
> Try a dry mineral makeup foundation to use in place of powder. Lightly dust over liquid foundation for a fresher finish.

or pale pink that you can apply first to the entire eyelid. This neutral color will be your base or "prep" color. Apply it evenly and lightly to the eye-lids, blending up to the brow. If you have droopy or puffy eyelids, keep this light, neutral color matte without shine or irridescence.

To define your eyes, you need to know what shape they are. If you look yourself straight into your own eyes in the mirror and can see the lower edge of your upper eyelids, then you have a lidded European eye and will have many options for colors and multicolor effects. If you look straight ahead and see only the color part of your eye and the pad of your eyelid, then you have a Mongolian-shaped eye that won't carry a lot of shadow but needs to be defined around the lash line.

> ### Lashes Tip
> For a special event when you want to look your most fabulous: Using tweezers and your 5X mirror, add two individual demi-eyelashes to the outside corner of each upper eyelid. Use temporary adhesive and set them right into the lash line, allowing a few of your own lashes to separate them. Wait until the adhesive has dried to clear before applying mascara. They will blend in with your own lashes and add just enough length to be glamorous and look like they are natural, even when looking closely. For dark brunettes only, use the black medium-length flair lashes. For all other hair colors use brown medium-length lashes. If your lashes are sparse and short, you may want to use the short length. Never pull on a lash held in place with dry adhesive; it will take with it any lashes connected to it, leaving bare spots. Remove when bathing or washing your face and the adhesive is wet and softened.

Look at the color of your eyes. All the colors you see are generally safe to use in defining your eyes. Think again about light and dark and the power they have to reshape and define. We will use the darker color to "set back," soften, or delete falling eyelids or puffiness, or fullness above the eyes. If your personal color palette is warm tone, you will use a light-to-medium brown or fawn shade, depending on how much drama you are trying to create. If your palette is cool tone, you will use a grey, grey-brown, or dove shade of shadow. Using a sponge-tip or bristle shadow brush, load the brush with your darkest color. Use each color of shadow separately. Do not mix colors on the brush; this will "muddy down" the shadow color and take away definition.

For lidded European eyes, start from the outside corner of the brow bone and work across towards the center. Gently blend the edges until the shadow appears soft and there is no apparent edge.

For Mongolian eyes, use the darkest of your brown or gray shadow; load a fine-tip brush (or you can turn your sponge-tip applicator onto its pointed edge for definition). Apply shadow to the lower lash edge. Stay very close to the eye edge, going through the lashes, applying the heaviest concentration at the outside corner. Blend.

Mascara Application

Apply two coats of mascara to upper and lower lashes, waiting a minute or two in between coats. Drying time allows you to build up and thicken your lashes. Don't be afraid to use the tip of the wand to bring out tiny lashes close to the inner eye. Lift upward as you apply. When lashes are lifted and perky, eyes are more open and prominent.

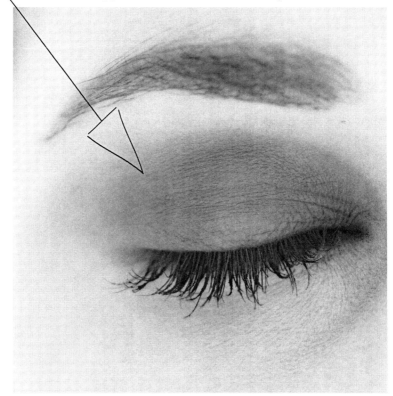

Lips

Lipstick is the number-one selling item in the multibillion dollar cosmetic industry. It is the first piece of makeup most young women purchase, and most mature women a generation ahead of them won't leave their home without it. Your lips are the heart of your smile and every word you speak. They have more movement than your nose, eyes, chin, and brows so they attract more attention. It is a shame to leave them bare. Leaving lips bare is leaving your face unfinished, as if you forgot something. Lipstick provides needed color to the face as it moisturizes your lips. When properly done, lips can bring your other facial features into balance, whereas overdone lips tend to attract so much attention you can't see beauty in the face—just lips. Using the proper tools and techniques you can make a wide face appear more narrow, thin lips appear fuller, tooth discoloration appear less noticeable, and your overall look appear balanced.

Make your determination: Look at your lips in the mirror. Check to see if the outside corners of your mouth match up. If your top lip tapers down and stops before it reaches the outer corner of the bottom lip, or if your bottom lip does not quite reach the outside corner of your upper lip, then you have one lip smaller

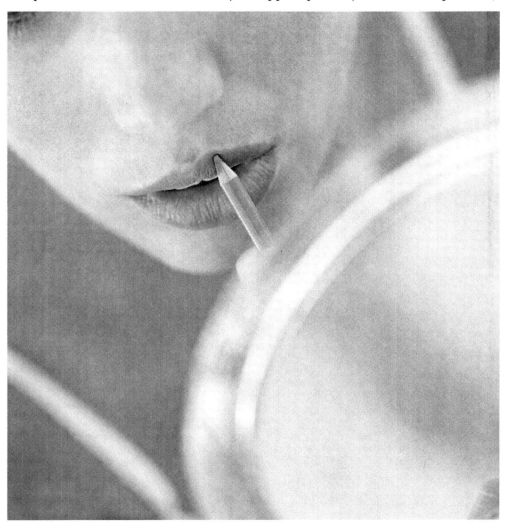

than the other — or mismatched lips. If your face is full or large, your mouth may appear small, whereas a thin, small face may cause lips to appear full. In any case, there are adjustments that can easily be made with a lip liner.

Your lip-liner should be a color that is natural to your face. Stay away from lip liner colors that are too brown or dark. We want to perfect the symmetry of the mouth by gently extending or minimizing your natural lip line where necessary. You will work right along the natural lip edge. This can be tricky if you have a double lip edge or a very rounded shape to your lips. Be careful not to draw too far away from the lip edge onto the skin.

For Men

The goal here is to have everything you need within easy reach so grooming is fast and flawless. Make sure you have an organized area in a bathroom drawer or medicine cupboard for all your grooming tools. These items are your own personal grooming kit and should not be shared with family members.

These are "must-haves":

- small scissors
- eyebrow comb/brush
- razor
- lotion or cream for shaving
- hair brush
- comb
- tweezers
- hand mirror
- after-shave skin conditioner

All personal toiletry items should be handy and kept in a clean, convenient place.

Eyebrows

Often I work with men who have never had one minute of groom training. Not one lesson. They simply had to shave so they found the easiest method, period. And for some men, whether it's fear of acting feminine, or not knowing where to go to get the information or just not realizing they need grooming, that's where it ends. So, starting from the beginning, in order to make you look your most handsome, we need to recognize your good features. On a scale of 1–10, rate your physical characteristics, 10 being best, no need for improvement, 1 being you realize it needs lots of help.

- Your hairline
1 2 3 4 5 6 7 8 9 10
- Hair Thickness and Amount
1 2 3 4 5 6 7 8 9 10
- Your Hair Color
1 2 3 4 5 6 7 8 9 10
- The Tone in Your Neck
1 2 3 4 5 6 7 8 9 10
- Eyebrow Shape
1 2 3 4 5 6 7 8 9 10
- Teeth
1 2 3 4 5 6 7 8 9 10

Skin

For years I have worked on the most beautiful faces in the world, but the ones I found memorable and truly beautiful were the ones that had imperfections. A nose slightly longer than what would be considered perfect, a tooth slightly turned, or eyes with a certain character — these imperfect features are what create charm and remind you of your ethnicity or inherited family features. A truly beautiful woman or man is groomed, authentic, and interesting. Cosmetic procedures such as injected lips and tight face lifts are evident and usually send a message of insecurity. Nothing is sexier than someone who is confident in their own skin. This takes grooming, not surgery. Invest time and effort in grooming, keep makeup simple and stay free of resentments and grudges, and you are on your way to authentic beauty.

Let's talk about food again. Here's an article from my column, "All Health's Breaking Loose."

Daily Bread — Take your Glasses

From my Column

There's nothing like a good loaf of bread. We've all been told we should eat whole wheat bread and, for some of us, that's where the criteria begins and ends. But there's a lot more to selecting a good quality loaf of bread. Too much wheat in the system can trigger a myriad of problems in the gut, unexplained rashes, skin conditions, and sinus problems and other ailments. Switching from whole wheat to spelt, barley, millet, oat, or rice may give your system a chance to recover from the stress wheat may be bringing to your body. But whatever grain you chose, the most important thing is to take your glasses with you to the market. You'll have to get past the pretty picture of the old flourmill or sun-kissed golden grain on the plastic wrapper and read the label.

Back in the fifties, scientists figured out how to completely strip all the nutrients out of a grain of wheat, leaving a lighter, more finely ground flour that subsequently could rise higher — it was fluffy and soft. They gave it names like "Wonder" and Moms were thrilled — it seemed softer and better! But what was left behind was pretty much useless to man or animal. With the germ and bran gone, only the endosperm was left, which has the least nutritional value. But we liked it so much, we got on board with words like "enriched," thinking it had been made "better" as the word suggests. However, in reality they were putting back only a very small part of what had been taken away in the first place. So the first rule: if it says "enriched" or "unbleached enriched" wheat (or other) flour, it should be skipped altogether. Stone ground can also represent basic wheat flour unless it says "whole wheat" or "whole grain" on the back label. And "made with whole grains" does NOT mean it contains whole grain unless it says so on the back label[2]. Yep, you're gonna need your glasses.

As you read the ingredients list, remember, the ones at the beginning of the list are used in the largest quantity. So if items like whole wheat, whole barley, or whole oat are near the bottom of the list, there's not going to be very much whole grain included. Watch for the sugar content and how high up on the list it is — hopefully not in the first five. Breads that contain oats are going to require more sweetening and raise the calorie content (ever tasted plain processed oatmeal? Eew). But at all costs, avoid high fructose corn syrup. It's the big kahuna of junk foods and your body was not designed to store this type of garbage.

We may think we're buying the "good stuff," or the expensive name brand, but price and packaging has nothing to do with quality. It can't be good if all its "good stuff" has been modified or removed. We weren't consulted when manufacturers figured out genetic modification would be very profitable for them, even if it endangers our health. Unless the bread has the certified organic symbol on the label, you have no way of knowing how much real grain (grain NOT genetically modified) was used. The biotech industry genetically modifies (GM) not only the grains in bread, but pasta, cereal, granola bars, and many of the other foods we eat. As much as 70% of the foods sold nationwide—in your town and mine — are GM, says Jeffrey Smith, spokesperson for the Institute for Responsible Technology. It's simple: foods that resist frost, bugs, and have a longer shelf life

---

2. Edited by Bushuk, W. and Rasper, V.F. <u>Wheat Production, Properties and Quality.</u> London: Blackie Academic and Professional, 1996

mean more profits. Critics of GM foods say Americans are being used as guinea pigs in an experiment without the benefits of proper assessment or control. Experts say that parts of the proteins in GM soy are identical to known allergens, and one of their concerns is that if parts of the gene inserted into the GM grain end up transferring into the DNA of human gut bacteria, this could produce its own potentially allergenic protein[3]. Your own intestines could begin to produce a risky, allergenic protein that makes you sick.

Sadly, the risk for food allergies is higher now than ever before--especially in children. We hear a lot about allergies in the news, but rarely are they mentioned in connection with genetically altered food. In 1999 researchers at York Laboratories in the UK were alarmed to discover that adverse reactions to soy products had skyrocketed 50% over the previous year. Their spokesperson said, "We believe this raises serious new questions about the safety of GM foods." In 2002, Canada began a study to see if GM foods posed a danger, and within a year abandoned the study saying it was just too difficult to monitor.

Many countries have banned GM foods, but here in America we are surrounded by them[4]. Currently there are no standardized methods to evaluate the safety of GM foods. Wow — they're in our markets, we feed them to our families, and no one really knows what the effects could be!

You can limit your family's exposure to GM foods by buying bread and other products that are certified organic or that say "non-GMO." You can also avoid the "nasty seven," or the seven crops that have been genetically engineered: soy, corn, cottonseed, canola, Hawaiian papaya, and small amounts of zucchini and crookneck squash. This includes snack foods that contain cottonseed or canola oil, sweets with corn syrup, and soy lecithin in chocolate.

John Boyles, MD, an Ohio-based allergy specialist says, "I used to test for soy allergies all the time, but now that soy is genetically engineered, it is so dangerous that I tell people to never eat it — unless it says organic." The more we petition our local grocery stores to carry organic bread and other products, the sooner we'll have a good selection of reasonably priced organic foods to choose from.
End of Column

IF IT'S NOT ORGANIC, IT'S NOT GOOD ENOUGH FOR YOUR BODY.

And lastly, avoid calcium sulfate and calcium propionate; they are mold inhibitors that cause irritability, sleep loss and allergic reactions. Look for organic,

---

3. Institute For Responsible Technology. "Genetically Engineered Foods May Cause Rising Food Allergies." 2007 May. www.organicconsumers.org/articles/article_5296.cfm

4. Hanyona, Singy. "Another Poisoned Chalice in Africa." Norfolk Genetic Information Network. 15 May 2008. www.ngin.tripod.com/200802e.htm

whole-grain bread with understandable ingredients and at least 3 grams of fiber per serving. Whole grains are loaded with fiber — which lowers your risk for diabetes, heart disease and digestive and breast cancers. Complex grains are also great for lowering your cholesterol. They're loaded with trace elements such as zinc, magnesium, selenium, copper and iron, as well as B vitamins and vitamin E.

- Try grains other than wheat.
- If it says "enriched" it should be ditched.
- Watch for the certified organic symbol.
- Avoid high-fructose corn syrup, calcium sulfate, calcium propionate, other preservatives and additives.
- Combine bread only with vegetables, not protein or fats.

It takes just a little knowledge to choose a really wonderful loaf of bread. You don't have to be a scientist … you just have to take your glasses.

Five-Star Maintenance

Throughout my career I've spent countless hours grooming celebrities—the biggest and the brightest, from coast to coast and continent to continent. I've seen true beauty radiating naturally and real ugliness polished up to be attractive. I may have seen it all—hissy fits and outbursts, kindness under pressure, grace, nastiness, inflated egos and down-home sensibilities. On a regular basis I have fielded comments like, "Isn't it exciting to meet and talk with —————? (Fill in your favorite "A" lister here. What is he/she like?" Our fascination with celebrities has become toxic. What is of most importance at this point is YOUR life coming into balance. Isn't your own happiness and productivity more important than that of someone whose job it is to entertain you? Some are lovely people and some are cranky and self-centered — just like the rest of the world, and that's it. Any energy spent on wondering about someone else's life is wasted energy. You need that energy to heal and maintain your own body and life. Let's allow them to do what they do best and focus our attention on meaningful events. The world would be a better place if the paparazzi were out of a job. So, as we've talked about before, habits are more easily replaced than dropped so, as you walk past the tabloid stand, leave those stars alone and count YOUR own stars…

Your goal is to accrue five stars every day. Keep a running tally in your head. You're already eating whole, organic super foods in proper combination, so here is a simple daily checklist to keep you feeling and looking great — with very little trouble.

Five Stars a Day

Your Goal is to acrue at least 5 stars a day.

2 stars for being "sugar-free"
2 stars for exercising and stretching (at least 45 minutes)
1 star for meditation
1 star for eating in combination with something from the "A" list included
1 star for being meat free. (Be aware of the days you have animal protein and fish so you're not consuming meat daily.) You'll find balance by spacing these days out.
1/2 star for being dairy-free
1 star for having a shot of wheat grass (1 or 2 oz. 2-3 times per week)
1/2 star for having a sauna, massage, or facial (no more than once per week)
1 star for drinking 10 ounces or more of fresh-squeezed vegetable juice

On a perfect day you'd accrue 10 stars and be in the absolute pursuit of health and beauty. "10 Star" days will reverse your aging process and keep you in the center of the path that leads to wellness and beauty. These days are a treat to your body — the more of them you have, the leaner, younger, and more youthful you'll feel and look. "10 Star" days help you to remain disease free, as your body is healing, renewing, and rebuilding on these days. I hope you feel fantastic. You have to love these days — your body does!

Between 5 and 10 stars is beautiful and will help you maintain or continue to lose weight — great job!

Let the Rain Wash Away the Years

Remember when you were a kid — how special a rainy day was? There was nothing like tipping your head back and letting the raindrops pat your face. If you opened your mouth you might even be able to catch a few on your tongue. When, along the way growing up, did the rain become a hassle? Was it when we hurried to get the groceries in from the car without getting wet, stressing over ruined makeup, or — heaven forbid — our hair went straight and flat?

Recently I met with a group of boot campers for an outdoor training session in the rain. As we did our opening salutation (shown in Week Four), we came to the posture #13, also shown in Week Four, with our hands on the lower back, head tipped back and chest lifted up toward the sky. For a moment, we all had our faces up, catching the rain on our cheeks. It got very quiet. It gave us a chance to re-feel a childhood moment.

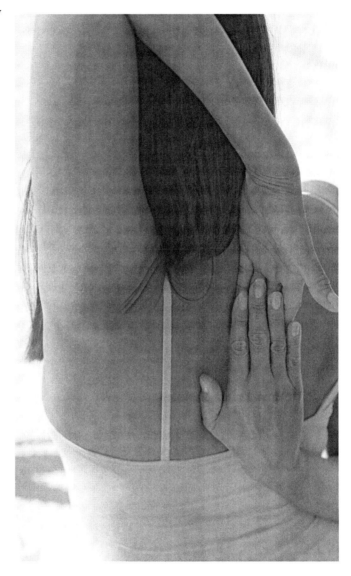

Every cell of your body has intelligence, and that intelligence has memory. As we revisit positive childhood sensations, we exercise our cellular memory. An ageless mind is curious and open to new ideas, like a child. An ageless mind can stay in the moment without regret of the past or fear of the future[5]. In that small moment of catching a little rain in the face, those boot campers exercised so much more than their bodies. They exercised their child-like spirit and opened themselves up to a new possibility — maybe it's okay to let my face get wet. New possibilities are where we find even more of our own potential.

But first, they had to be there. They had to show up. Waking up to a rainy day, knowing it's cold outside and you're going to get muddy—well, you have to dig down pretty deep to find the determination to get yourself out the door to exercise. But, once that decision was made, it was easy. And because they were there, they not only had a great workout, they regained a youthful awareness

---

5. Chopra, Deepak and David Simon. Grow Younger, Live Longer. New York: Harmony Books, 2001.

for their body in that quiet moment when the rain fell on their cheeks. The mind and body connect through our awareness. In that connection, energy flows freely throughout the body and THIS wonderful moment is when the body heals itself efficiently. Healing allows the aging process to slow down or even stop.

Like them, you have exercised your childlike spirit by trying elements of this program that are new to you. You have opened yourself up to new possibilities. You have stood strong when faced with temptation and turned away from old toxic habits. The pay off will continue to surprise you, and there is more of it to come as the "Authentic You" progresses. Good for you! Congratulations!

When the body "shows up" and the mind "opens up" it is the perfect scenario to train your body to be the best it can be.

Next time you're out in a rainy day, tip your head back and see if the rain washes away a few years.

We can only learn about our own body by listening on a deep personal level to all it tells us. If we take the time to stay in tune with all our systems, we can discern truth from error. When we know the truth about what really brings us health, we will have the body we have always wished for — fit, lean, pain-free, and strong. The experience we have been sharing — your private, individual Wellness Boot Camp — will put you into the "flow" of health if you allow it to. Some of these practices may have been new to you, but as you allow them to become habits, you apply your personal truths to yourself. You become authentic. The "Authentic You" lives effortlessly in the flow of health. These are your personal truths, and as they resonate within you, it gets easier and easier to stay in the flow — you begin to radiate health.

> We cannot teach people anything; we can only help them discover it within themselves.
> — Galileo

Dealing and Healing

As your life unfolds, you are experiencing one continuous transformation. Your body is evolving, and there's no reason to expect decline. Your body is the one machine that improves with use. How wonderful! Rather than expect your hair to gray and your body to stiffen, wrinkle and become fragile as others' bodies around you are changing, stay connected to how you feel in your own body. Stay open to the idea that you will have good health your entire life. Let your body demonstrate what it can do. Expect to have more vitality, more creativity and a stronger mental capacity as the years go on. Maturity of the mind and youthful vigor of the body are the ultimate combination. The quality of your life can increase according to your interpretations and choices.

> *For attractive lips, speak words of kindness.*
> *For lovely eyes, seek out the good in people.*
> *For a slim figure, share your food with the hungry.*
> *For beautiful hair, let a child run his or her fingers through it once a day.*
> — Audrey Hepburn

Your constant state of renewal never stops. It takes a few days for your stomach lining to replace itself, weeks for your liver to be entirely rebuilt and in about one years time, your entire body will have been completely made new — each and every cell has been replaced[6]. You are renewing and healing at every moment and may go long periods of time where all you see is improvement in your body. If those around you are turning gray or getting wrinkles — it is of no concern to you. Assuming you will do the same will hasten your aging process. We become what we expect to become. where aging is at a standstill. Don't concern yourself with whose hair is gray or which of your friends have wrinkles. Expecting yourself to do the same will only expedite your aging process. We become what we expect to become. You are on your own unique, individual path.

With a refreshed view of your circumstances, heightened awareness of your body, and habits that fortify and renew you — you are becoming timeless. You helped write this book with your journaling. Your intuitive observations will lead you to personal truth, and a body you admire that coincidentally looks great in jeans. And even better, you now have the tools to look and feel as good as you want to! I hope you re-read, study, and thoughtfully consider what both you and I have expressed in these pages. By keeping these concepts fresh in your mind, new powerful habits become part of you. You begin to want what you need and that is

---

6. Greenz. "Interesting Facts about How your Body Rebuilds Itself." Word Press. 5 May 2008. www.greenze.com/2008/08/interesting-facts-about-how-your-body-rebuilds-itself/

a reward all of its own. Your mind and body will work effortlessly in synergy — you just have to listen.

Your "Personal Boot Camp" is not ending; rather, new possibilites have opened up and what lies ahead is bright and beautiful. The "Authentic You" is just beginning.

You're "charting your own course"— and when you chart your own course, you write your own history. History is written all around you every day. This wellness experience is part of your history and you are creating it. Rather than just enduring the life that someone else has made for you, you've chosen a direction.

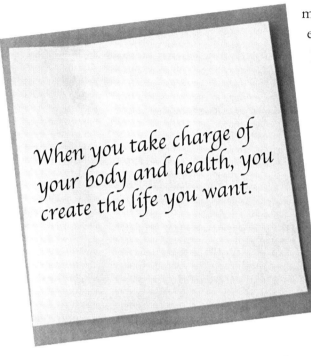

When you take charge of your body and health, you create the life you want.

When you choose a direction and dedicate yourself to it, you make history. When you listen to naysayers trying to convince you that it can't be done or get distracted by meaningless details, you endure history. When you allow outside forces to dictate your mood, you get the life that's given to you. But when you set your priorities and stick to them, you make history. There are an infinite number of possible histories out there, waiting to be lived by you.

Whatever your life has been up to this point doesn't matter. What counts is the history that awaits you in the future. You have chosen a powerful path. It's amazing to witness your own transformation.

If a client came to me and explained that cancer runs in their family and they would like to begin an anti-cancer program, this is the program I would put them on. If they asked for a weight loss program, this is the program I would put them on. If they asked for a cholesterol-lowering program, a plan to reduce their depression, anxiety, arthritis, or reduce their chance of becoming diabetic, or if they needed to balance their hormones and reduce PMS or menopause, yes — this program is how you achieve all of the above. You can gain control over your own health and thereby your destiny.

Here's what you've done:

I hope you feel great about your progress over the last seven weeks. Remember many of the wonderful changes that have taken place are on the inside of you.

You have reduced your risk of

• heart disease • cancer • diabetes • depression • asthma • infectious illness • Alzheimer's • arthritis

You'll notice improvement in

• headaches • irritable bowel syndrome • indigestion • acne • anxiety • mood swings • PMS • menopause • fatigue • foggy thinking • joint pain • immune function

Celebrate your renewal

• balanced hormones • lower cholesterol • slower rate of aging • youthful brightness to the skin • plenty of energy • creative ideas • contentment

This Week's Assignments:

- Work out a minimum of 4 times this week using all exercises consecutively, so the routine is fluid and smooth. Make sure you are including plenty of cardio this week, such as thirty minutes of walking or biking daily. Challenge yourself by adding push-ups in sets of ten and do 2–3 sets, or abdominal crunches in sets of 25, and do 3–4 sets.
- Meditate daily.
- Maintain eyebrows.
- Eat in proper combination.

New Goals:

- Purchase at least one makeup tool that you need to complete your personal kit.
- Practice facial highlighting.
- Pay special attention to blending in your makeup application.

Today's date _____

You're Invited

Join me for a

Special Celebration

Date: Today
Time: Commencing immediately
Place: My home

Contentment, peace, joy, good food, and well-being will attend me from this moment on.

No gifts please — I have everything I need.

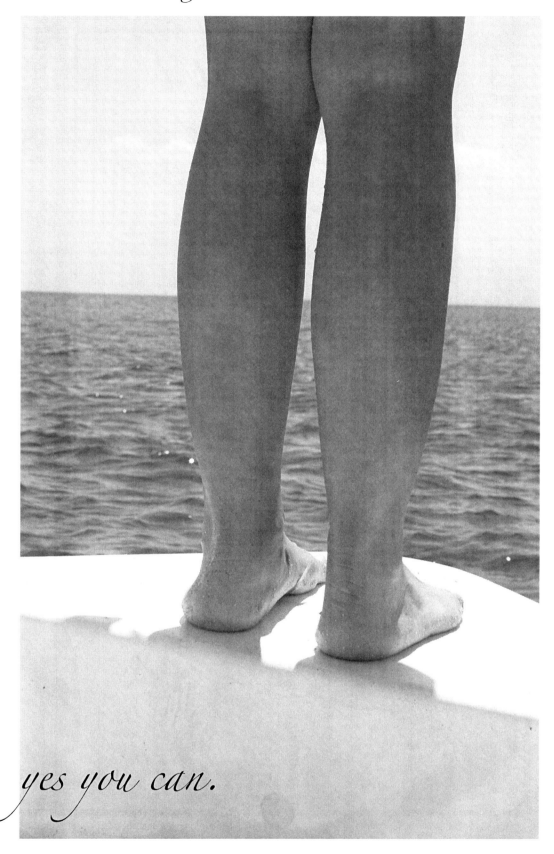

Appendix:

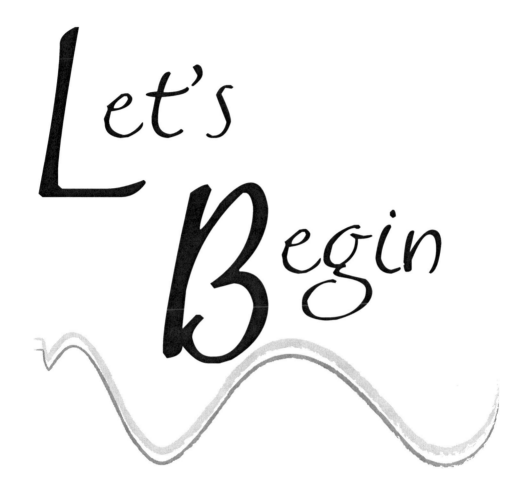

Let's Begin

Take this questionnaire and these measurements at the beginning, and throughout your wellness journey.

Questionnaire

Today's date_____

1. Do you have a compulsion to eat or drink certain foods? Circle those that apply: chocolate   breads   salty foods   fast food   coffee   sweets   soda   alcohol   other:_____

2. On a scale of 1 to 10, (10 being excellent with no concerns) rate your overall health: (circle)   1   2   3   4   5   6   7   8   9   10

3. With 10 being strong, energetic, pain free, calm and joyful, rate how you feel:
   1   2   3   4   5   6   7   8   9   10

4. Rate your level of stress. 10 being nervous, anxious, prone to tears, or depression, 1 being calm, content, and happy:
   1   2   3   4   5   6   7   8   9   10

5. Collectively rate the relationships in your life, 10 being fulfilling and peaceful, 1 being difficult, strained, or bothersome:
   1   2   3   4   5   6   7   8   9   10

6. Do you have pain in your body: never   occasionally   often   constantly

7. Tension in your body is usually stored in your: upper neck & shoulders   abdominal area   mid-back   low-back   head   other:_____

8. List injuries that limit your exercise performance_____

9. Do you feel you look older than your chronological age   younger than your age   age appropriate

10. Are you a worrier?   Y   N

We need accurate measurements.

Bust line: arms down by your sides, running the tape measure straight across the front of your chest

Bottom rib: run the tape measure straight across your lowest rib

Waist at the smallest point

Hip, stand with your feet together, measure at the widest area

Right arm: with your arms down, measure just under your arm pit check to see all of the tape is aligned horizontally

Be sure you have included the date. We will retake these measurements later on.

Today's Date _____

Bust_____

bottom rib_____

Waist_____

Hips_____

Rarm_____

Blood pressure:_____ (averaged a.m. and p.m. reading)

Cholesterol

HDL_____

LDL_____

Appendix:

Food Journal

To begin with, we need to get accountable. Make two copies of the food journal pages. Each week, record your daily food intake. Log your exercise, meditation, disposition, and food as accurately as you can through Weeks Two and Three. Clarity comes from reviewing your choices on paper. Enter your weekly totals at the end of the week. Beginning with Week Four, trust yourself and let your awareness keep you accountable.

Day 1

Day of the week_____ Date_____

Breakfast_____

Lunch_____

Dinner_____

Snacks_____

Water intake; circle one for each 8 oz. glass

* * * * * * * *

Emotionally, today I feel: _____
_____

Physically, today I feel: _____
_____

Meditation time_____

Exercise time_____

Wheat grass (if yes, check here)_____

Day 2

Day of the week_____

Breakfast_____

Lunch_____

Dinner_____

Snacks_____

Water intake; circle one for each 8 oz. glass

* * * * * * * *

Wheat grass, circle one for each single ounce shot

* *

Emotionally, today I feel: _____
_____

Physically, today I feel: _____
_____

Meditation time_____

Exercise time_____

Food Journal

Day 3

Breakfast_____

Lunch_____

Dinner_____

Snacks_____

Water intake; circle one for each 8 oz. glass

* * * * * * * *

Wheat grass, circle one for each single ounce shot

* *

Emotionally, today I feel: _____
_____

Physically, today I feel: _____
_____

Meditation time_____

Day 4

Breakfast_____

Lunch_____

Dinner_____

Snacks_____

Water intake; circle one for each 8 oz. glass

* * * * * * * *

Wheat grass, circle one for each single ounce shot

* *

Emotionally, today I feel; _____
_____

Physically, today I feel; _____
_____

Meditation time_____

Exercise time_____

Day 5

Breakfast_____

Lunch_____

Dinner_____

Snacks_____

Water intake; circle one for each 8 oz. glass

* * * * * * * *

Wheat grass, circle one for each single ounce shot

* *

Emotionally today I feel: _____
_____

Physically today I feel _____
_____

Meditation time_____

Exercise time_____

Day 6

Breakfast_____

Lunch_____

Dinner_____

Snacks_____

Water intake; circle one for each 8 oz. glass

* * * * * * *

Wheat grass, circle one for each single ounce shot

* *

Emotionally, today I feel: _____
_____

Physically, today I feel: _____
_____

Meditation time_____

Exercise time_____

Day 7

Breakfast_____

Lunch_____

Dinner_____

Snacks_____

Water intake; circle one for each 8 oz. glass

* * * * * * * *

Wheat grass, circle one for each single ounce shot

* *

Emotionally, today I feel: _____
_____

Physically, today I feel: _____
_____

Meditation time_____

Exercise time_____

Weekly Totals

Wheat grass shots

Mon Tues Wed Thurs Fri Sat Sun, (circle the days) — list number of wheat grass shots _____

Exercise time: Hours_____Minutes_____

Days of exercise_____

Total meditation time _____

This week I overcame: _____
_____

I am proud of myself for trying:_____

Next week I will be better at:_____
_____

Journal about difficulties here:

Foods_____
_____

Emotional Situations_____

Appendix:

Here are some recipes that may provide inspiration on how to really "eat well." Some are here because they offer foods you may not eat often but would like to try in a different way, and some are here to help you cook with more fresh, whole, super foods. There is no reason to measure or weigh to find portion size. Feelings of restriction do not exist with the vegetable recipes because you are cooking with what your body needs. Listen to your body and eat until you are satisfied. There are a few meat recipes included for those who wish, but portion size does need to be taken into consideration for those — meat should be eaten sparingly.

All ingredients in these recipes should be organic.

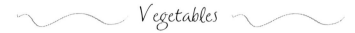

Tomato and Fennel Salad
Makes four 1-cup servings

Prep time is about 10 minutes. Heirloom tomatoes are great in this simple salad. They're at their peak in the summer months and worth seeking out at the Farmers Market or grocery store. Any will work well. Very low calories, zero cholesterol, 3 grams protein, loaded with fiber, vitamins C and A and potassium.

- 1 T. extra virgin olive oil
- 1 T. champagne vinegar or white wine vinegar
- ½ t. salt
- freshly ground pepper to taste
- 1 pound organic tomatoes cut into wedges
- 2 C. thinly sliced organic fennel bulbs
- ¼ chopped fresh parley
- 1/3 C. toasted pine nuts (see toasting tip below)

Whisk oil, vinegar, salt and pepper in a large bowl until combined. Add tomatoes, fennel, parsley and pine nuts. Toss to coat.

TIP: Toast pine nuts in a small dry skillet over medium low heat, stirring constantly, until fragrant and lightly browned, 3-5 minutes.

Jicama Summer Salad
Makes 2 servings

A crunchy, refreshing side dish or snack — takes minutes to prepare.

- 1 medium jicama, julliened small like matchsticks
- ½ C. small organic red onion, thinly sliced
- ¼ C. chopped fresh cilantro
- ¼ of a yellow bell pepper, thinly sliced (so it is compatible with jicama)
- juice from 1 lime
- coarse salt and fresh cracked pepper to taste

Combine all ingredients and toss. Best if served immediately, but will keep well if covered in the fridge.

Vegetables

Zucchini and Carrots With Green Onions and Dill
Makes 8 servings

A really good alternative to basic steamed vegetables — serve simply with roast chicken. If you are trying to lose weight save this recipe for later.

- 1 ½ to 1 ¾ pounds of organic zucchini, trimmed, coarsely grated
- 3 T. olive oil
- 1 ½ C. chopped green onions (about 6 large), divided
- 1 ½ pounds organic carrots (about 5 large), peeled, coarsely grated
- 4 T. fresh dill, snipped finely with kitchen scissors, divided in half
- 1 tablespoon organic butter

Roll up grated zucchini in large kitchen towel; press to dry.

Heat oil in deep skillet over high heat. Add 1 cup green onions and sauté 30 seconds. Add zucchini, carrots, and 2 tablespoons dill. Saute until vegetables are just tender, tossing often, about 8 minutes. Mix in remaining ½ cup green onions, butter and 2 tablespoons dill. Season to taste with salt and pepper.

Aromatic Herb Frittata with Arugula Salad
Makes 8-10 servings

8 large organic eggs
- ½ C. fresh marjoram leaves
- ½ C. Italian parsley
- ½ C. fresh basil
- ½ C. fennel fronds (tops)-optional
- 2 scallions thinly sliced
- 1 T. chopped fresh thyme
- 1 T. chopped fresh sage
- 2 T. unsalted butter for pan
- 1 C. arugula, sorrel or tender lettuce cut into thin strips
- 1 ½ t. red wine vinegar
- 1 ½ T. extra virgin olive oil
- 1 T. agave nectar

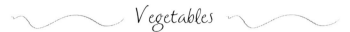
Vegetables

In large bowl, beat eggs and salt and pepper until frothy. Add ¼ C. each of marjoram, parsley, basil and fennel, and all of the thyme and sage until well combined.

Heat butter in an 8" or 10" skillet on stove on medium heat until almost browned. Add eggs and cook on medium until set, about 7 minutes. Hold a flat plate over pan and invert. Then slide back into pan to cook the other side until set, about 6-7 more minutes. Allow to cool for 10 minutes and cut into wedges.

In medium bowl combine remaining herbs with arugula or lettuce and toss in olive oil, vinegar and agave nectar. Serve alongside frittata.

Basil Vinaigrette Salad dressing
Makes about 1 2/3 cups

- 2 cloves garlic
- 3 T. basil chopped
- 2 T. chives, snipped finely with kitchen scissors
- 1 shallot finely minced
- 1 t. Dijon mustard
- ½ C. white wine vinegar
- 1 C. extra virgin olive oil
- freshly ground sea salt and black pepper

Crush the garlic, basil, chives, and shallot until like a paste. Add to food processor along with mustard, vinegar, salt and pepper. Mix thoroughly. Drizzle the oil steadily into the processor while running until all ingredients are emulsified.

Saute'ed Goat Cheese and Tomato Salad with Micro Greens
Makes 4 servings

- ¼ C. fine whole-grain dried breadcrumbs
- Sea salt
- Freshly ground black pepper
- ½ teaspoon water
- 1 organic egg

Vegetables

- 4 rounds fresh goat cheese
- 4 thick, ripe beefsteak tomato slices or nice heirlooms if available
- 2 teaspoons olive oil plus more for the salad
- 2 C. micro greens
- Vinaigrette made of ½ cup each olive oil and white balsamic vinegar, wiith 1 t. finely chopped dill, 1 clove very finely chopped garlic, freshly cracked salt and pepper and a splash of agave nectar. Whip with a fork.

In a shallow bowl mix the breadcrumbs with salt and pepper to taste. Add the water and work it in with your fingers to lightly moisten the crumbs. In another small, shallow bowl, beat the egg with a fork just until blended. Dip one flat surface of each goat cheese round in the egg, and then in breadcrumbs, patting the crumbs in place. Repeat on the other flat surface, leaving the sides of the rounds uncoated. Place the breaded goat cheese rounds on a small parchment paper-covered baking pan or plate. Refrigerate the rounds for about 15-20 minutes. Place the tomato slices on 4 serving plates. Season with salt and pepper — drizzle with the vinaigrette

Heat a large nonstick skillet over moderately high heat. Add the 2 tablespoons olive oil. When the oil is almost smoking add the cheese rounds, one coated side down. Cook until lightly browned, about 45 seconds, then gently turn (I find 2 forks works best) and cook on the second side until just BEFORE the cheese gets soft, about 45 seconds longer, depending on the thickness of the rounds. Place a cheese round on each tomato slice.

Mound the micro greens on top of the cheese, dividing evenly. Drizzle a bit of the vinaigrette around each plate and serve immediately. Do not dress the micro green directly, they wilt down quickly.

Baked Stuffed Zucchini
Makes 6-8 servings

This recipe is from my mother. In her hand written cookbook she referred to the "food chopper" rather than processor. Zucchini is loaded with vitamin C, magnesium, beta-carotene, potassium and riboflavin. It is high in fiber, which helps to lower cholesterol. The vitamin folate found in summer squash is need by the body to break down a dangerous disease promoting metabolic byproduct

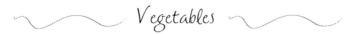

called homocysteine. Squashes have anti-cancer properties. Studies on their juices have been shown to prevent cell mutations or cancer-like changes.

- 8 small to medium organic zucchini
- 2 medium organic onions
- 1 clove garlic
- 12 sprigs fresh parsley
- 3 T. olive oil
- 1 C. cooked and drained organic Swiss chard or spinach (about 10 oz)
- 1 T.. fresh or 1 t. dried oregano leaves
- 1 ½ t. salt
- Fresh cracked pepper to taste (1/8 t. or so)
- ½ C. grated Parmesan cheese
- 3 organic eggs beaten
- 2/3 C. dry organic whole-grain breadcrumbs

Cook zucchini in boiling water for 5 minutes. Drain and cool. Cut in half lengthwise. Scoop out center pulp; discard seeds, reserve meat leaving ¼ shell all around. Chop onions, garlic and parsley in blender or food processor. Sauté in oil. Put zucchini pulp and chard (or spinach) through food chopper or in blender. Drain off excess liquid. Add to onion mixture and sauté. Add seasonings and cheese; mix well. Add eggs and crumbs and blend. Sprinkle zucchini shells lightly with salt. Fill with pulp mixture and sprinkle lightly with more breadcrumbs. Bake in slow oven, 325 degrees until golden – about an hour. Can be made ahead and frozen. Thaw to room temp, cover and bake, removing the foil for the last 10 minutes.

Garlic Sauté

*Substitute any vegetable you like for any of those listed below.

Makes 4 servings.

- 2 1/2 C. Brussels sprouts with loose outer leaves removed, cut in half (about 1/2 pound)
- 2 1/2 C. yellow squash or zucchini, cut into 1/4-inch slices (about 1/2 pound)
- 1 large tomato (or 2 small), diced
- 4 teaspoons extra virgin olive oil

Vegetables

- 1 teaspoon minced garlic
- 1 tablespoon shredded or grated Parmesan cheese

Put Brussels sprouts, squash, and a couple tablespoons of water in a microwave-safe dish and microwave on HIGH until vegetables are lightly cooked. Drain well. Add oil and garlic to large nonstick frying pan or skillet and heat over medium heat for 1-2 minutes. Stir in the Brussels sprouts, squash, and tomato. Sauté for a few minutes, or until vegetables reach desired doneness. Sprinkle Parmesan cheese over the top and serve.

Vegetables Glazed With Balsamic Vinegar
Makes 4 servings

- 3 T. olive oil
- 1 clove finely chopped garlic
- 1 organic red bell pepper, cut into ¼ inch strips
- 1 organic yellow bell pepper, cut into ¼ inch strips
- 1 medium organic onion, thinly sliced
- 2 organic zucchini, trimmed, cut crosswise into ½" thick rounds
- 2 organic yellow summer squash, trimmed cut crosswise into ½" thick rounds
- 2 T. balsamic vinegar
- 1 tablespoon agave nectar

Heat oil in heavy large non-stick skillet over medium high heat. Add peppers, garlic and onion. Sauté until beginning to soften, about 4 minutes. Add zucchini and yellow squash and sauté until tender, about 9 minutes. Add vinegar to skillet and boil until liquid is reduced to glaze and coats vegetables, 2-3 minutes. Season to taste with salt and pepper. Transfer to platter and serve.

Roasted Root Vegetables
Makes 8 servings

- 4 slim organic carrots peeled and sliced diagonally into 1 inch pieces
- 10 organic baby turnips, peeled, halved
- 10 organic baby brussel sprouts (do not cut them)

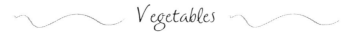
Vegetables

- 4 large organic parsnips, peeled, trimmed, and cut diagonally into 1 inch thick slices
- 1 medium organic onion, trimmed, peeled, halved – cut each half into quarters
- 1 large organic beet, peeled and cut into thick wedges
- 1 kohlrabi bulb, peeled and cut into thick wedges (can also use cabbage)
- 1 organic celery root, trimmed and halved, halves cut crosswise into 1 inch thick slices
- 1 whole head of garlic, separated into cloves, unpeeled
- 2-3 sprigs fresh organic rosemary, sage or thyme
- Sea salt
- Freshly ground black pepper
- Extra virgin olive oil
- 2 T. balsamic vinegar

Preheat the oven to 400 degrees. Put the cut vegetables, garlic and the herbs in a large baking dish. Season with sea salt and black pepper, balsamic, drizzle generously with olive oil, and toss them with your hands to coat them evenly. Place the baking dish in the preheated oven and cook, stirring the vegetables occasionally, until they are tender and golden brown, about 45 minutes. Serve as a side dish with a protein and green vegetables.

Red Pepper and Garlic Dip
Makes 6 servings (1 cup)

A nice hors d'oeuvre pairing fresh vegetables with a simplified version of rouille, the spicy red pepper and garlic sauce that typically accompanies French fish soups.

- 2 large garlic cloves
- ½ C. diced, drained, roasted red pepper from jar
- ½ teaspoon red wine vinegar
- ¼ teaspoon cayenne pepper
- ½ C. organic mayonnaise
- ½ teaspoon fresh oregano or pinch of dried oregano

Vegetables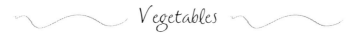

Prepare colorful fresh vegetables like carrot, celery and jicama sticks, yellow bell pepper strips, baby grape tomatoes and boiled baby potatoes. With food processor running, drop garlic in and mince. Scrape down sides of bowl. Add roasted pepper, vinegar, oregano and cayenne and process until mixture is a almost a smooth puree. Add ¼ cup mayonnaise and process using on/off turns just until combined. Transfer sauce to a small bowl. Mix in remaining ¼ cup mayonnaise. Season to taste with freshly cracked sea salt and pepper. Cover and refrigerate for 30 minutes (can be prepared a day ahead — keep refrigerated).

Place dip in center of platter. Arrange vegetables around dip and serve.

Saute'ed Mushrooms
Makes 2 servings

- 1 lb. fresh sliced shiitake, Portobello, and button mushrooms, (mixed according to your favorites — if you prefer, use all one kind)
- 3 T. Chicken or vegetable broth with 1 t. whole wheat or other flour stirred in
- 2 cloves finely chopped garlic
- 2 T. Extra virgin olive oil
- 2 T. Braggs liquid aminos
- 2 T. fresh rosemary
- salt and pepper to taste
- parmesean cheese to taste

Chop garlic and let it rest as you remove stems from mushrooms and slice. Heat olive oil in a skillet. Add garlic and allow to soften for 2-3 minutes. Whisk in broth with flour added and Braggs aminos. Add mushrooms and cover for three minutes. Add the rosemary, salt, and pepper, and continue cooking uncovered for 5 minutes or until desired tenderness.

Serve over brown rice, fish or chicken, or as a side dish.

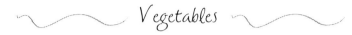

Vegetables

Cucumber, Radish, and Mint Salad
Makes 8 servings

- 8 kirby or 3 English cucumbers (organic, seedless)
- 2 bunches radishes
- 2 bunches scallions
- ½ C. white wine, champagne, or raspberry vinegar
- ¾ C. olive oil, walnut oil, or sunflower seed oil
- 1 T. agave nectar or honey
- 1 C. chopped fresh mint leaves
- salt and pepper

Peel and thinly slice the cucumbers. Cut the radishes into thin slices. Cut scallions on the diagonal and toss in with the cucumbers and radishes. Combine the vinegar, oil, and agave nectar. The dressing should be tart. Toss vegetable in the dressing. Right before serving toss the vegetables in salt and pepper and sprinkle with mint leaves; toss again.

Navy Beans and Chard
Makes 4 servings

- 2 T. oil
- ½ onion, sliced and quartered
- 1 large red bell pepper, sliced and quartered
- 2-3 garlic cloves, minced
- 5-6 C. chopped Swiss chard (pack lightly to measure)
- 2 C. well drained, cooked navy beans
- ½ C. cut corn
- ¼-½ C. chopped cilantro
- 1 t. seasoned salt (or to taste)
- ½ t. cumin powder
- ¼ t. kelp granules or pepper

For best results, chop all vegetables first. In large skillet, heat oil. Stir in onion, red pepper, then garlic; sauté 1 minute. Stir in chard; sauté 1 more minute. Stir in remaining ingredients and just heat through.

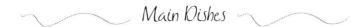

Main Dishes

Lemon and Herb New Potatoes
Makes 6 servings

- 2 lbs. new potatoes
- 2 finely minced cloves of garlic
- 1 t. freshly cracked sea salt
- cracked pepper to taste
- 1 lemon rind, finely grated plus the juice
- 1 ½ t. mustard
- 4 T. olive oil
- 2 T. chopped fresh chives
- 1 t. chopped fresh parsley
- 1 or 2 finely chopped green onions

On a baking sheet rubbed with olive oil, roast 2 pounds new potatoes or fingerlings with thick slices of onion until tender.

Meanwhile prepare ingredients. Whisk in the order given allowing extra whisking time to the olive oil addition. Mix the green onions in just before pouring over hot potatoes. Toss into potatoes gently and serve warm.

Vegetable Sauce
Makes about 2/3 cup

Great tossed over broccoli, green beans, spinach, peas or any favorite vegetable. Can be used as a sauce over brown rice as an entrée. Versatile and fast with lots of options to make vegetables special.

- 1/4 C. honey
- 2 T. onion, minced
- 1/4 C. organic butter
- 1 t. thyme, crushed
- freshly cracked sea salt and pepper, to taste

Combine all ingredients in a small saucepan and bring to a boil; cook 2 minutes. Toss with vegetables of choice and serve hot.

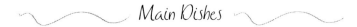

Main Dishes

Whole Wheat Turnover Pastry Dough
Makes 18 6-inch turnovers

The whole wheat flour in this recipe may be exchanged for spelt flour, brown rice flour, or other flour of your choice.

- 3 1/2 C. whole wheat flour
- 1/4 C. safflower oil
- 1/2 C. water
- 1/3 C. almond or rice milk
- 3 T. maple syrup
- 1 1/2 t. salt

In a large bowl, place the flour and drizzle in the oil. Using your fingers, work the two together until it forms a crumbly mixture. In a small bowl, place the remaining ingredients, and whisk well to combine. Add the wet ingredients to the flour mixture, mix well, and with your hands form it into a ball of dough. Transfer the dough to a floured surface. Divide the dough in half. Roll out one half of the dough thinly, cut eighteen 5-inch circles, and set them aside. Gather up the scraps, add the scraps to the remaining half of dough, roll out the dough thinly, and cut eighteen 6-inch circles. Fill the 6-inch circles of dough with up to 1/3 cups of desired filling. Wet the edges of the circles of dough with water, place the 5-inch circles of dough on top of the filling, press down around the edges of the dough to seal, and then crimp the edges with a fork. Use a spatula to carefully transfer the filled turnovers to 2 non-stick cookie sheets and bake at 350 degrees for 15-20 minutes or until lightly browned. Serve the turnovers hot or cold. Allow them to cool completely on racks before wrapping them individually in aluminum foil to preserve freshness. They can also be frozen in airtight containers after baking for later use.

Garden Veggie Turnovers
Makes 9 6-inch turnovers

Kids love these. They're a great way to train kids to enjoy vegetables. Variation: other vegetables may be used in the turnovers, such as peppers, tomatoes, broccoli, cauliflower, peas, greens, beans, etc. Use what you love to create your favorite turnover.

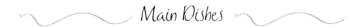
Main Dishes

- 3/4 C. onion, finely diced
- 3/4 C. carrot, finely diced
- 1/2 C. celery, finely diced
- 2 T. olive oil
- 1 1/2 C. red skin potatoes, scrubbed & cut into 1/2-inch cubes
- 1/2 C. zucchini, finely diced
- 2 t. garlic or more to taste
- 3 T. freshly chopped parsley
- 2 T. brown rice flour or Parmesan cheese
- 1 T. freshly chopped thyme
- 1/4 t. salt and ¼ t. pepper, freshly cracked
- 1/2 recipe of Whole Wheat Turnover Pastry Dough (enough for 9 turnovers)

In a non-stick skillet, sauté the onion, carrot, and celery in olive oil for 3 minutes. Add the potatoes, zucchini, and garlic, and sauté an additional 8-10 minutes or until vegetables are tender. Add the fresh herbs, nutritional yeast, salt, and pepper, and stir well to combine. Taste, adjust seasonings as needed, and set aside to cool. Prepare the dough for the turnovers. Then cut the 5-inch and 6-inch circles of dough as described in the turnover pastry dough recipe. On each of the prepared 6-inch circles of dough, place 1/3 cups of the vegetable filling. Wet the edges of the circles of dough with water, place the 5-inch circles of dough on top of the filling, press down around the edges of the dough to seal, and crimp the edges with a fork. Use a spatula to carefully transfer the turnovers to a non-stick cookie sheet, and bake at 350 degrees for 15-20 minutes or until lightly browned. Serve the turnovers hot or cold. Allow them to cool completely on a rack before wrapping them individually in aluminum foil to preserve freshness. They can also be frozen in an airtight container after baking for later use.

Spaghetti Squash and Meatballs
Makes 4 servings

One of my family's favorites and simple to prepare.

FOR THE SQUASH
- 2 organic spaghetti squashes (about 2 pounds each) halved lengthwise and seeded
- 1 T. extra virgin olive oil

Main Dishes

- Salt and freshly cracked pepper

FOR THE SAUCE
- 2 T. extra virgin olive oil
- 4 cloves garlic finely chopped
- 2 T. organic tomato paste
- 2 cans (28 ounces) crushed organic tomatoes with basil
- 1 T. fresh or 1 t. dried oregano
- Coarse salt and freshly cracked black pepper

FOR THE MEATBALLS
- ½ C. fresh organic whole grain breadcrumbs
- ½ C. grated parmesan-reggiano cheese (and more for serving)
- ¼ C. chopped fresh parsley
- ¼ C. chopped fresh thyme
- 2 large cloves very finely chopped garlic
- 1 pound ground turkey
- 1 large egg
- ¾ t. coarse sea salt
- Freshly cracked black pepper
- 3 T. extra virgin olive oil for skillet

To prepare the spaghetti, preheat the oven to 400 degrees. Drizzle cut sides of squash with oil and season with salt and pepper. Place cut sides up on a baking sheet. Bake until soft to the touch, about 1 to 1 ¼ hour.

To prepare the sauce, heat the oil in a saucepan over medium high heat. Add the garlic and cook, stirring with a wooden spoon for about 1 minute. Add the tomato paste and cook, stirring, for an additional 3 or 4 minutes to brown slightly. Stir in the tomatoes and the oregano, season with salt and pepper. Bring to a boil and reduce to a simmer. Cook stirring occasionally, until thickened, about 20 minutes. Keep warm over low heat.

To prepare the meatballs, in a medium bowl, stir together the breadcrumbs, parmesan, parsley and garlic with a wooden spoon until combined. Add the turkey, egg, salt and pepper, and mix with your hands until well combined. Form mixture into 1 ½ inch balls.

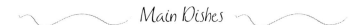
Main Dishes

Heat the olive oil in a large non-stick skillet over medium high heat. Working in 2 batches, cook the meatballs until evenly browned, turning often, about 6 or 7 minutes. Repeat with remaining meatballs. Transfer meatballs to the sauce and simmer until cooked through, about 10 minutes.

When the squashes are cool enough to handle, scrape the flesh of each squash with a fork into spaghetti looking strands, and place into a large bowl. Serve topped with meatballs and sauce, and sprinkled with cheese if desired.

Ginger Beef and Kale
Makes 4 servings

- 1 pound organic filet mignon thinly sliced
- 2 T. finely grated fresh ginger
- 5 garlic cloves minced
- 1 large onion, finely grated, about 2/3 C.
- ¼ t. smoked paprika
- 2 small hot dried red chiles, crumbled
- ¼ t. coarse sea salt
- 1 t. extra virgin olive oil
- 1 bunch organic kale (1 ½ pounds) stems discarded, leaves cut into 3 pieces each and rinsed.
- ½ C. homemade or organic canned beef broth
- ½ t. freshly ground black pepper

Combine beef, ginger, garlic, onion, paprika, chiles, and salt in a bowl, making sure the beef is well coated. Heat oil in a large sauté pan over medium high heat. Add beef mixture and cook, stirring frequently, until lightly browned, 2 to 3 minutes. Stir in kale and cover, reduce heat to medium low. Cook stirring occasionally until wilted, about 5-7 minutes. Uncover and raise heat to medium high. Add stock and cook, stirring and scraping bottom of pan, for 1 minute. Season with pepper.

Chicken Breasts With Sage
Makes 4 servings

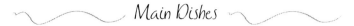

Main Dishes

- 2 large all natural, organic boneless, skinless chicken breasts, filleted lengthwise and gently pounded with a mallet so they are thinner and more tender
- Salt and freshly ground black pepper
- Juice from 3 lemons
- 6 T. extra virgin olive oil
- 40 fresh sage leaves
- 4 T. organic unsalted butter
- 4 lemon wedges for garnish

Season the chicken breasts with salt and pepper. Place them in a casserole dish. Add the lemon juice, half of the oil, and the sage leaves. Turn the chicken to coat evenly, cover and set aside at room temperature for 30 minutes.

Heat a large skillet on medium low heat. Add butter and the rest of the oil. When hot and bubbly, take each piece of chicken out of the marinade (reserving marinade and sage leaves) and place in skillet. Cook until golden brown, about 5 minutes. Turn the chicken breasts over, then take the sage leaves out of the marinade and add them to the bottom of the skillet. Cook another 5-7 minutes until breasts are cooked through. The sage should get nice and crispy. If it begins to burn, remove it from the pan and set aside. Remove the chicken breasts and sage leaves and cover loosely with foil while you make the sauce.

Return the pan to medium heat. Add the reserved marinade and stir with a wooden spoon, loosening up brown bits from the bottom of the pan. Let the sauce boil until it reduces to a thick syrupy sauce. This takes a minute or two. Pour the sauce over the chicken. Garnish with lemon wedges. Serve immediately.

The chicken should be tender enough to eat with a fork. It is a simple, fresh tasting dish that is great when served with asparagus or any favorite green vegetable.

Garlic Dijon Salmon
Makes 4 servings

- 4 (6 ounce) salmon fillets
- 1/3 C. Dijon mustard
- 1 T. olive oil for preparing pan plus 2 T. for cooking onions and garlic

Main Dishes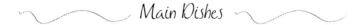

- 4 large cloves garlic, thinly sliced
- 1 red onion, thinly sliced
- 2 teaspoons chopped fresh tarragon (or 1 t. dried)
- Salt and pepper to taste

Preheat oven to 400 degrees. Rub a 9" x 13" inch pan with olive oil. Heat olive oil in a saucepan on low. Add the garlic and onion slices. Cook on low, stirring occasionally until caramelized, about 25 minutes or until desired tenderness. Arrange the salmon skin side down in the prepared pan, season with salt and pepper and lightly coat with the Dijon mustard.

Bake 20 minutes in the preheated oven, or until salmon is easily flaked with a fork. Arrange onions and garlic on top of salmon, garnish with tarragon and serve.

Salmon with Lentils
Makes 4 servings

- ½ pound French green lentils (lentilles du puy)
- ¼ good olive oil, plus extra for salmon
- 2 C. chopped organic yellow onions
- 2 C. chopped organic leeks, white and light green parts only
- 1 t. fresh thyme leaves
- 2 t. kosher salt
- ¾ t. freshly ground black pepper
- 1 T. minced fresh garlic
- 1 ½ C. chopped organic celery (4 stalks)
- 1 ½ C. chopped organic carrots (3 carrots)
- 1 ½ C. homemade chicken stock, or good canned organic broth
- 2 T. tomato paste
- 2 T. good red wine vinegar
- 1 T. agave nectar
- 4 (8 ounce) center-cut salmon fillets, (preferably wild Alaskan) skin removed

Place the lentils in a heatproof bowl and cover with boiling water. Set aside for 15 minutes, then drain. Meanwhile, heat the oil in a sauté pan - add the onions.

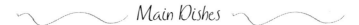 Main Dishes

Leeks, thyme, salt and pepper and cook over medium heat for about 10 minutes, until the onions are translucent. Add the garlic and cook for 2 more minutes. Add the drained lentils, celery, carrots, chicken stock and tomato paste. Cover and simmer over low heat for 20 minutes, until the lentils are tender. Add vinegar, agave nectar and season to taste.

Preheat the oven to 450 degrees. For the salmon, heat a dry ovenproof sauté pan over high heat for 4 minutes. Meanwhile, rub both sides of the salmon fillets with olive oil and season the tops very liberally with salt and pepper. When the pan is very hot, place the salmon fillets seasoning-side down in the pan and cook over medium heat without moving them for 2 minutes, until very browned. Turn the fillets and place the pan in the oven for 5 to 7 minutes, until the salmon is cooked rare. Spoon a mound of lentils on each plate and place a salmon fillet on top. Serve hot.

> The lentils can be made separately and used as a side dish for just about anything. Lentils are a complete protein and digest very well with meats and veggies. They are one of the most powerful sources of protein available. Not only do lentils help lower cholesterol, they are a special benefit in managing blood-sugar disorders since their high fiber content prevents blood-sugar levels from rising rapidly after a meal. They are high in vitamin and minerals, fat free and low in calorie — just 230 calories per cup of cooked lentils!

Herbed Frittata

- 2 T. butter, or more if needed
- 2 T. minced chives or onions
- 1 1/2 C. fresh herbs and greens, all carefully cleaned and dried, then torn into small pieces
- 12 large eggs
- 6 T. rice milk, almond milk (or divide so 3 T are the milk and 3 T are cream)
- 1 tablespoon finely ground wheat flour
- ¾ C. grated cheese
- Freshly ground salt and black pepper

Thoroughly butter the bottom and sides of an 8-inch nonstick skillet. If 2 tablespoons are not sufficient, use more butter. Place the pan over low heat; when the butter becomes warm, add chives or onions. Heat gently, just until they give

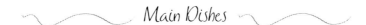

Main Dishes

off a little fragrance. Add the herbs and greens and, if necessary, a little more butter. Stir so that all the flavors mingle.

While the greens are heating, beat the eggs, milk, flour, cheese and a little salt and pepper into a large bowl.

Preheat the oven to 300 degrees. Prepare the greens as above and transfer to a buttered 13" x 9" baking dish. Beat the eggs, milk, flour, cheese, and pepper in a large bowl and pour over the greens. Bake for 15-16 minutes.

Flourless Cheese Souffle'

Makes 4 servings

Serve as a protein with a side or salad or veggies.

- 2 T. butter, softened
- 6 large organic eggs, separated
- 1 pinch cayenne pepper
- 1 shallot finely grated
- ½ t. freshly grated nutmeg
- Salt
- Fresh ground black pepper
- 4 oz organic cream cheese, softened
- 1 ½ C. finely grated organic Gruyere or Swiss cheese

Preheat oven to 425 degrees. Coat a 6-cup soufflé dish with the butter. In a mixing bowl, combine the egg yolks, shallot, cayenne pepper, nutmeg, salt and pepper. Beat with a wire whisk until light and fluffy. Add the cream cheese and grated cheese and whisk until smooth and well combined. In another bowl, beat the egg whites until peaks are almost stiff. Gently fold the egg whites into the cheese mixture. Spoon into the greased dish and place on baking sheet. Bake 10 minutes. Reduce heat to 400 degrees and bake an additional 15 minutes.

Serve immediately.

Parmesean & Grilled Onion Frittata

- 1 organic red onion, cut into 8 equal size wedges
- 1 organic yellow onion, cut into 8 equal size wedges
- ½ teaspoon salt

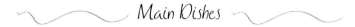

- ¼ teaspoon freshly ground black pepper
- ¼ C. olive oil
- 10 medium organic eggs
- ¼ C. organic heavy cream
- 3/4 C. freshly grated organic Parmesan cheese
- 2 T. unsalted organic butter
- 1 teaspoon finely chopped fresh rosemary
- 1 teaspoon finely chopped fresh sage

Preheat oven to 350 degrees. In a large bowl, combine onions and olive oil and toss to coat well. Preheat a grill pan over high heat. Arrange onion wedges on grill pan and cook until browned and tender underneath, about 5 minutes. Turn onions over and cook until very tender and brown, 7-8 minutes more. Brush with more oil as needed. In a large bowl, beat eggs and cream. Stir in ½ cup cheese, salt and pepper until smooth. In a 10-inch braiser or oven-proof frying pan over medium low heat, melt butter. Add rosemary, sage and cook, stirring, 1 minute. Poor egg mixture into pan and fold gently to combine rosemary and eggs. Arrange grilled onions over top of eggs. Sprinkle with remaining cheese.

Transfer pan to oven and bake until frittata is golden brown and puffy, about 12 to 15 minutes.

Spinach Frittata
Makes 6-8 servings

Frittatas are a versatile egg dish much like an omelet. They are a great way to use any leftover vegetables you have, like asparagus, red pepper, mushrooms, etc. Try adding different herbs — experimenting is part of the fun and a great way to find what your family loves. If inverting it out of the pan intimidates you, pour all ingredients into a baking dish and bake at 300 degrees for 15 minutes, checking for doneness and if needed bake 5 minutes more.

- 2 lbs. fresh organic spinach
- 2 T. extra virgin olive oil
- 1 finely chopped medium onion
- 1 T. fresh finely chopped chives (if not available, use a larger onion)
- 8 large organic eggs

Main Dishes

- ¼ C. Parmesan reggiano cheese
- ½ grated sheep's milk cheese such as Cacio di roma (or this can be replaced with the same amount of Parmesan)
- ¼ C. Parmesan reggiano cheese
- Freshly cracked salt and pepper

Bring 6 quarts of water and 2 T. sea salt to boil. Plunge spinach in and cook for 2 minutes. Drain and put into ice bath to preserve green color. Drain in colander or roll in clean kitchen towel to remove water. Chop finely on cutting board.

In a 9-inch sauté pan heat olive oil until hot, add onion and stir until clarified and soft, about 5 minutes. Meanwhile in separate bowl, beat eggs until frothy, then add remaining ingredients to mix well. Pour into buttered non-stick skillet and cook over medium heat until bottom is set — about 5 minutes. Place a plate over skillet and invert out of pan; slide back into skillet to cook the other side, about 5 minutes more.

Veggie Burgers
Makes 6 servings

Get your groove on at the next burger/dog party with these healthy, tasty burgers. Ingredients should be organic-use vegan versions. These measurements are estimates!

- 1 can beans or lentils
- your favorite veggies such as carrots, zucchini, or broccoli
- 1/2 C. salsa
- 1 Tablespoon sesame oil
- 1 Tablespoon vegan Worcestershire sauce
- 1 C. rolled organic oats
- 1/4 C. cornmeal

Blueberry Ginger Bellini
Makes 2 servings

Not only refreshing and beautiful but loaded with anthocyanidins (antioxidants).

- ½ C. mashed blueberries

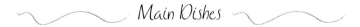

Main Dishes

- garlic powder
- onion powder
- salt and pepper
- 1/4 C. barbecue sauce

Drain and rinse your beans or lentils (black beans, red, or pinto would be good, too). Puree in food processor. Put pureed beans in mixing bowl.

Put your veggies in the food processor — about 2 cups. After processing there will be about 1 cup. Add this to the mixing bowl. Process rolled oats in the food processory to create a powdery grain. Or for more texture, skip this step.

Add all ingredients to mixing bowl and combine. If mixture is too wet to make patties, add cornmeal. Form into 6 patties and salt and pepper the tops. Place on a lightly oiled cookie sheet and bake at 350 degrees for about 30 minutes.

Ratatouille

Makes 4-6 servings

- ½ C. olive oil
- 4 cloves garlic, minced
- ¼ C. chopped parsley
- 1 T. thyme leaves
- small bunch basil
- 1 eggplant, cut into 1/3-inch-thick slices
- salt to taste
- 2 zucchini, sliced
- 1 large onion, sliced into rings
- 2 C. sliced fresh mushrooms
- 1 yellow bell pepper, sliced
- 1 red bell pepper, sliced
- 2 large tomatoes, chopped
- grated Parmesan cheese

Preheat oven to 350 degrees. Coat bottom and sides of a 1 1/2 quart casserole dish with 1 tablespoon olive oil.

Main Dishes

Heat remaining olive oil in a medium skillet over medium heat. Sauté eggplant until tender, turning once and set aside. Do the same for peppers, then set aside — if desired, slip the skins off when cooled. Sauté garlic until lightly browned. Mix in parsley and thyme, add to eggplant. Season with salt to taste, keeping peppers separate.

Spread eggplant mixture into an even layer across bottom of prepared casserole dish. Sprinkle with a few tablespoons of Parmesan cheese. Spread zucchini in an even layer over top. Lightly salt and sprinkle with a little more cheese. Continue layering in this fashion, with onion, mushrooms, bell pepper, and tomatoes, covering each layer with a sprinkling of salt and cheese. Add only one light sprinkling of basil mid-way through.

This takes about 15-20 minutes to make. Bake in preheated oven for 45 minutes. Use remaining basil leaves for garnish. Delicious served with brown rice.

Drinks

- 1 T.. minced ginger
- Juice of ½ lemon
- Agave nectar, xylitol, or stevia — sweeten to taste

Mash all ingredients and add 2 cups blueberry (or pomegranate) juice. Let steep for at least 5 minutes. Strain. Divide between 2 champagne flutes and top with sparkling mineral water.

Iced Mint White Tea
Makes 4 servings

Loaded with flavonoids (antioxidants) and vitamin A.

- ½ C. fresh mint leaves
- 3 white tea bags
- 3 T.. agave nectar
- 4 C. boiling water

Combine and let steep for 5 minutes. Remove tea bags. Refrigerate until really cold. Divide among 4 large ice-filled glasses. Garnish with a stalk of lemongrass.

Loaded with flavonoids (antioxidants) and vitamin A.

Cantaloupe Crush
Makes 2 servings

- 1 C. cantaloupe cubes
- 1/3 C. pineapple chunks
- ¼ C. orange juice
- ½ C. peaches
- 1 pinch stevia or t. honey or agave nectar to taste
- 3 ice cubes

Whirl all ingredients in a blender until smooth. Breakfast option or after-

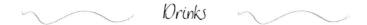

Drinks

noon pick-me-up. Replaces fruit so drink when stomach is empty.

Princess Lemonade
Makes about 3 cups

Just as Sleeping Beauty was awakened with a whiff of rosemary water, this herbal lemonade will awaken your senses as well.

- 1 ½ C. cold filtered pH balanced water
- 1 ½ C. agave nectar
- 1 ½ C. lemon juice (meyer lemons are best)
- Finely grated rind of one lemon
- 3 sprigs of rosemary
- ice cubes
- cold mineral water, sparkling or flat

Combine the water and agave nectar in a saucepan. Bring to a boil over high heat and cook for about three minutes. Remove from heat and add the lemon juice, rind and rosemary. Refrigerate for 2 hours and strain into a storage container.

To prepare one serving: drop crushed ice into a glass. Fill about half full with lemon syrup. Top off with flat or sparkling mineral water, garnish with a fresh strawberry or sprig of mint, stir and drink.

Tropical Smoothie
Makes 2 servings

- 1 mango, peeled and seeded
- 1 papaya, peeled and seeded
- ½ C. fresh strawberries
- 1/3 C. orange juice
- 4 -6 frozen pineapple juice cubes

Make ice cubes with pineapple juice ahead. Put all ingredients in a blender and process until smooth. A refreshing, low-calorie pick-me-up or after workout drink.

Drinks

Fruit and Veggie Cooler
Makes 2 servings

- 1 C. apple juice (unfiltered is best)
- 1 C. sliced sweet apples
- ¼ C. apple sauce
- ½ C. sliced carrots
- ½ C. peeled and sliced cucumber
- dash of nutmeg or cinnamon — optional
- 1 C. ice — optional

Put all ingredients into blender and blend until smooth. Give it time to get through all the vegetables. A great "wake up" beverage and perfect replacement for coffee.

Acknowledgments

Thank you to my parents, Bess and Chet Johnson, who taught me to trust in the power of the human body. They were the original alternative healers.

Thank you to my many wellness campers and clients over the years, whose dedication and desires have shown me that the human spirit is capable of altering the body. Raindrops and perspiration rolling down their smiling faces will be forever etched in my memory. And thank you to the readers of my column, "All Health Is Breaking Loose," whose kind responses underscore the fact that we all on some level are in pursuit of feeling better.

Thank you to David Blasucci for believing in me and spurring me on to completion. Your encouragement and support helped me overcome the odds and finish this project. Your "stick with it" attitude was always what I needed. I could not love you more than I do.

To my children — Cheston, Thomas, Sadie, and Samuel — your laughter and comedic genius keep me on my toes. Thank you for being productive and happy as you set out to make the world a better place. Because of how you manage your lives, I have been free to devote the years of my life that it took to create this program and finish this book. You are the funniest and most brilliant people I know. You, along with Jessica, Shalee, Sophie, Bronx, and Joseph are the reason I wrote it.

Tami Marshall, April Clive, Ann "Boo" Curtis, and Nicole Carlson — thank you for reading draft after draft and always contributing with insightful commentary. Your concern for this project truly gave me the courage to keep "swinging for the fences." Tyraysha Peterson, thank you for your help with illustrations and photography. Janet Crowley, thank you for the assistance with the illustrations and for letting me paint "Steve McQueen's Dog Has A Glass Eye" on your dining room wall — just for fun. Little did we know at the time it would end up in a book!

Thank you to Patti F. Smith Esq., my dear friend and attorney, for always looking after me. Your genius has blessed my life many times. And to Steven C. Kalas M.Th., thank you for graciously sharing your gift with words.

And finally, from the deepest part of my heart, earnest appreciation goes to Amanda Crabtree whose patience and competence brought this book to life. Your fresh approach and many technical gifts have produced the look and feel of the book I was hoping for. I will be forever grateful for your organizational skills, graphic design "chops" and optimism that have seen me through to the end of this project. Neither of us knew the scope of this project from the outset and you have continually surprised me with your dogged determination to bring it to completion. With all your talent and patience, you are capable of anything!

Thanks to all of you — you are treasures to me. I am so blessed.

Love & health,

Loa

For more products, services, and
booking information visit Loa at *gotoloa.com*.

Designed and typeset by Amanda Crabtree.

Breinigsville, PA USA
17 June 2010
240117BV00001B/1/P